South Slavic Women's Transgenerational Trauma Healing Through Oral Memory Practices

South Slavic Women's Transgenerational Trauma Healing Through Oral Memory Practices

Women War Crimes and War Survivors

Danica Anderson

LEXINGTON BOOKS
Lanham • Boulder • New York • London

Published by Lexington Books
An imprint of The Rowman & Littlefield Publishing Group, Inc.
4501 Forbes Boulevard, Suite 200, Lanham, Maryland 20706
www.rowman.com

86-90 Paul Street, London EC2A 4NE

British Library Cataloguing in Publication Information Available

Library of Congress Cataloging-in-Publication Data Available

ISBN 978-1-66693-791-6 (cloth)
ISBN 978-1-66693-792-3 (ebook)

I dedicate this book to the Novi Travnik, BiH Kolo Sumejja Women War Crimes and War Survivors, especially the Kolo Sumejja leader, Susana Koric, who hosted me with grace no matter the situation. The support given to me by family, from both my daughter Dayo Vice (Dayana Marija Anderson) and my son Marko Joel Anderson, is extraordinary. In all, it is my mother, Zorka Medic Borkovich, concentration camp survivor, to whom I dedicate this book.

Contents

Acknowledgments ix

Chapter 1: South Slavic Women's Transgenerational Trauma Healing 1

Chapter 2: Invisible 19

Chapter 3: Social Memories 27

Chapter 4: Maternal Fright 47

Chapter 5: Female Social Justice: Oral Memory Traditions Kolo 73

References 97

Index 117

About the Author 125

Acknowledgments

My greatest appreciation to Susana and Nihad Koric, who hosted me for over two decades while I was doing my research and informed trauma treatment. The Kolo Sumejja women in Novi Travnik, BiH, are the real experts on healing trauma and have my gratitude. My family, Dayana Marija Vice and Marko Joel Anderson, supported me with deep love. Dayana Vice, I am so thankful for your theater arts social engagement treatments with the Kolo Sumejja women.

Chapter 1

South Slavic Women's Transgenerational Trauma Healing

My kolo informed trauma clinical practices take place in the Middle Canton of the mountainous region in the Bosnia Hercegovina town Novi Travnik with South Slavic Muslim women survivors of war crimes and war. The underlying reason for the decades of clinical work on South Slavic transgenerational trauma is clear—what can be done about the trauma wounds, how is the transgenerational trauma suffering healed? The path is in the women war survivors' narratives and stories that continue to provide firsthand experience and insight into the challenges and realities of Eastern Europe and the Balkan region.

Arriving in 1998, I witnessed the aftermath of the Balkan War (1991–1994) and the devastating impact it had on Novi Travnik's munitions factory. Despite the efforts to repair and rebuild, the town faces ongoing economic hardship, which in turn fueled issues such as corruption, fraud, human trafficking, prostitution, and the presence of mafia brotherhood groups.

Many of the women war survivors remarked that the war never ends and that it began long ago. Moreover, the aftermath of the war contributes to domestic violence and nonstate torture, political strife, and increasing ethnic divisions exacerbating the challenges confronting the community. The pervasive poverty and subsequent brain drain, where many individuals choose to leave the country in search of better opportunities, further complicate the region's recovery and development.

By highlighting the long-lasting effects of war and the complex socioeconomic dynamics the women war survivors' meme "the war never ends" literally continues to impact the region. By shedding light on these challenges, the women war survivors contribute to a deeper understanding of the ongoing struggles in the aftermath of the Balkan War.

SOMATIC NEUROBIOLOGICAL PSYCHOLOGICAL AND MEMORY SCIENCE IN NARRATIVES

The narrative herstory of South Slavic Muslim women survivors of war crimes and war is brimming with somatic neurobiological psychological and memory science roots. One would assume these women war survivors had postgraduate education. However, they are a motley group where due to World War II some of the elders didn't attend school past the second grade and/or the Balkan War interrupted their generations' education. I found that their herstories speak to deep consciousness and relationships in regard to healing transgenerational trauma through their Slavic oral memory traditions and practices adapted to their geographic location and environment.

When I began researching and tracing when the transgenerational trauma took hold, certainly, it is after a century of wars in the former Yugoslav region. It revealed two distinct groups of South Slavic Muslim women war survivors who lived in close proximity to each other during the Balkan War in Bosnia. Despite their geographical proximity, the women in these groups experienced different forms of war trauma: one group directly experienced war crimes, while the other group faced indirect trauma resulting from the effects of the war. The nuances are invaluable for healing and researching transgenerational trauma inclusive of culture. Human suffering arises from wounds both physiological and invisible. Trauma wounds from grief, loss of loved ones, and being humiliated, shamed, or raped are not readily visible.

The visible trauma wounding I felt when I first arrived at the old Sarajevo airport in 1998, militarized with US forces, induced a need to home in to specific groups. The different forms of war trauma experienced by the two South Slavic communal collectives of Muslim women living in close proximity during the Balkan War can have a profound impact on their collective memory and individual memory accounts. Traumatic experiences, especially of an extreme nature such as war crimes, rape, and other forms of violence, can leave lasting imprints on the psyche and shape the way individuals and communities remember and recount their past.

Collective memory is influenced by both personal and shared experiences, as well as by cultural and historical contexts. Traumatic events can evoke strong emotional responses and lead to the encoding of memories that are vivid and enduring. However, the way these memories are constructed and expressed can differ based on the type and severity of trauma experienced.

For women war survivors who endured different forms of war trauma, their memory accounts of the past may vary significantly. The nature of traumatic experiences, such as direct experiences of war crimes or indirect experiences of war trauma, can influence the way these memories are processed, stored, and recalled. Women who suffered extreme trauma, like rape war trauma, may have particularly complex and unique memory accounts, as such experiences can profoundly impact their sense of self, identity, and relationships.

Understanding and acknowledging these differences in memory accounts is crucial for providing sensitive and effective trauma support and healing. Recognizing the diversity of experiences and the varying ways trauma manifests in memory can inform tailored interventions and therapeutic approaches. It is also essential to approach the study of these memory accounts with cultural sensitivity and respect for the survivors' narratives, as they hold valuable insights into the psychological and sociocultural effects of war trauma.

By recognizing the significance of individual and collective memory in shaping the experiences of women war survivors, researchers and practitioners can gain a deeper understanding of the complexities of trauma and contribute to more comprehensive and empathetic approaches to healing and recovery (Fisher 1996; Sarkissian 2021).

The women war survivors' herstories guided the informed practices intended to prevent transgenerational trauma to explore and analyze the narratives and accounts provided. It was simply through taking into consideration the specific forms of trauma the women survivors of war experienced and how they moved from survivorship to healing through the framework of their Slavic oral memory traditions. Examining their lived experiences and the way they remember and interpret the past sheds awareness on the impact of trauma on individual and Slavic collective memory. However, the women war survivors are only asked about their victimization.

WAR TRAUMA MYTHIC NARRATIVES AND MEMORIES

The unique perspectives and experiences of these women affords a deeper acknowledgment of the complexities of war trauma and its effects on memory. It recognizes that different levels of trauma shape individual and collective narratives in distinct ways, and by examining these nuances, a more comprehensive understanding of the impacts of war trauma, including rape war trauma, is achievable.

By exploring the Slavic oral memory traditions of two groups of South Slavic women who experienced different forms of war trauma, a picture emerges of how these women construct, store, and share their memories in relation to somatic psychological healing practices. Their interviews are the space and place of herstories—narratives that provide insight into healing transgenerational trauma among the women war survivors in 2000 and 2022. This results in an extensive archive under Kolo Sumeja Women (KSW), along with relevant Slavic-oriented literature such as Bahtijaragic and Pim (2015) and Hunt (1989).

Through the kolo informed trauma psychological treatment of these women and their interviews, it became evident that their recollections, which form the core of their South Slavic oral traditions, exhibit characteristics aligned with megalithic propensities within mythic narrative somatic psychology discourse. There exists very little research and material regarding how women heal transgenerational trauma, let alone South Slavic women war survivors. This observation aligns with previous studies by Anderson (2015b), Cowan et al. (2021), and Goettner-Abendroth (2012).

A notable similarity between memory recollections and mythic narrative somatic psychology discourse is the emphasis on discovering meaningfulness. The memory narratives of South Slavic women who have survived war and war crimes are rooted in tacit knowledge, representing their maternal life experiences past and present. This tacit knowledge is associated with a biological epigenetic process referred to as maternal ecosopy, described by Wheeler (2006b). Epigenetics, a form of cellular memory, informs us about how environmental factors have our genes react while each one of our cells responds differently. It is a complex system, along with the epigenetic modulation dynamics that tell us that we can control the health of our genes and our bodies' response to stress and trauma.

The Slavic term Moist Mother Earth and the Slavic matrilineal tradition are housed in ecosopy. Ecosopy signifies a physiological atmosphere in which one can breathe normally without aid, similar to the process of pregnancy. The mythic somatic psychological narratives of past generations and of these present-day survivors function as a maternal ecosystem that continues to hold great meaningfulness for women who have survived war.

The decades of studying the women war survivors arise with efforts that deepen the understanding of the relationship between Slavic memory recollections, mythic narratives, and somatic psychological healing in the context of South Slavic women who have survived war and war crimes. Exploring the interplay between these elements contributes to a broader comprehension of the significant impact of Slavic oral traditions on the healing process.

There are three profound elements in the South Slavic women war and war crimes somatic psychological discourse in the maternal ecosystem healing of transgenerational trauma. The first is the interactions with the environment. The second element is the embrace of social engagements, social relations moving toward growth and potential lived to their fullest and acquiring and knowing when to employ vital survival-resiliency skills. The third is the mother's life experiences standing center as an inheritance. The South Slavic women survivors of war and war crimes cite their inheritance as the narrative of the flesh which the fetus interprets as the possibilities of becoming—their potential (Wheeler 2006b; Porges 2007; Anderson 2015b; Christie and Pim 2012).

In terms of neuroscience and the neurobiology of trauma, the drivers of Slavic cultural behaviors are a bewildering array of forces in constant motion (Anderson, Blood and Honey Icons: Biosemiotics and Bioculinary 2012). Ranging from epigenetic inheritance, developmental plasticity, and the niche construction of Slavic culture right down the microbiome transfers—the gut and Slavic food and agrarian way of life are the significant role of genes in the process of evolving—healing from what needs to be healed in the environment.

TRANSGENERATIONAL TRAUMA AND EVOCATION

The South Slavic Muslim women war crimes and war survivors continue to heal their transgenerational trauma through evocation. The significance of evocation and the South Slavic earth-based practices does not lie in how they fix themselves or people. Nor was it a step-by-step instruction. Instead, I find memory, the South Slavic oral memory practices, a catalog of tacit knowing that is conjured through remembering, in the active verb tense as opposed to remembering past tense.

Basically, it is the concept that "I continue to learn" that is crucial in my development and implementation of my clinical kolo-informed trauma practices. Healing trauma centers on each person's tacit knowing—knowing without being taught to search for solutions within us evoking the healer-shaman (Anderson, Blood and Honey South Slavic Women's Experiences in a Modern Day Territorial Warfare 2015).

The healing process experienced by South Slavic Muslim women survivors of war crimes and war is characterized by the use of evocation and earth-based practices. Evocation, in this context, refers to the act of calling forth and invoking healing practices within oneself and the surrounding environment. It is not a prescriptive, step-by-step process but rather an exploration of memory and the use of South Slavic oral memory practices.

Since the focus is not on "fixing" oneself or others, it is about tapping into the deep reservoir of personal and cultural memory—maternally inclusive. By engaging with these memory practices, individuals can access their tacit knowing, a form of knowledge that is innate and intuitive, without the need for explicit teaching. This tacit knowing becomes a valuable resource in the search for solutions and healing.

The implementation of clinical kolo-informed trauma practices is informed and shaped by the understanding and application of South Slavic oral memory practices. These practices emphasize the significance of memory in the healing process and serve as a foundation for the development and implementation of therapeutic approaches.

In this healing paradigm, each person's unique journey is central, and the focus is on evoking the inherent healer within themselves. The concept of the healer-shaman is evoked, highlighting the role of the individual as an active participant in their own healing process.

By integrating memory, evocation, and the wisdom of oral traditions, the South Slavic Muslim women survivors of war crimes and war find a pathway toward healing trauma that is rooted in their own lived experiences and cultural heritage. This approach recognizes the importance of personal empowerment and the use of internal resources for healing and transformation.

WE ARE FLESH

The Bosnian women, in their close-knit sisterhood community of South Slavic cultural traditions, possess deep meaning in their cultural behavioral customs and relationships and, through this meaning, their vital survival and flourishing skills are well established (Hubbs 1993). The Slavic Balkan culture and oral memory traditions establish rituals that are somatic and movement-based, incorporating human intuition and tacit knowing that give rise to perception (Polanyi 1948, 29; Anderson 2015a; Ilieva and Shturbanova 1997).

The *soma*, Slavic "we are all flesh" is the Slavic Moist Mother Earth for the Balkan and Slavic women as in prehistoric artifacts and images, presents the Slavic women's perception of the world at hand. Joan Marler's (2003) book *The Body of Woman as Sacred Metaphor* explores the prehistory of Slavic culture during the pre-Indo-European period. Marler states that it is cultivation of a relationship with the entire natural world. Marler reports how rituals add inner coherence:

> Most of the anthropomorphic imagery is female, indicating the centrality of women's activities within the domestic and horticultural realms. In Gimbutas' view, a vast body of Neolithic symbolism reflects "a cohesive and persistent ideological system" expressing the religion of the Great Goddess. These symbols must be studied "on their own planes of reference, grouped according to their inner coherence." (Marler 2003)

For example, the plane of reference—the term "dual faith-Russian" for *dvoevire* is still highly regarded by the South Slavic women survivors of war crimes and war, and is influential in Balkan and Slavic cultures, especially on oral memory practices. It examples the continuing thread of women's tacit knowledge, a folk matriarchal culture in contrast to today's patriarchal religions (Hubbs 1993). These prehistoric oral memory rituals are still practiced but have adapted and evolved according to women's inner coherence in an escalating lethal patriarchal environment.

In the face of trauma, the female body must endure not only physical pain, but also the impact of the emotional pain as it is felt throughout the body. For example, female biological processes, such as menstruation, affect women's perception of their environment and experiences, with empirical evidence suggesting that during menstruation, pain is induced when viewing unpleasant images (Rhudy and Bartley 2010).

Note the biological and neurological processes work together, influencing the trauma victim either positively, as in the healing process, or negatively, as the victim suffers. It is not just the unpleasant images or/of horrific war trauma images. For thousands of generations, South Slavic women have recognized the importance of using body movements to connect, empathize, and eventually heal as a community. These oral memory rituals and movements are expressed in the Mesolithic folk round dance or gathering in a circle known as the *kolo* (Christie and Pim 2012; Anderson 2015b; Ilieva and Shturbanova 1997).

Investigating further, the South Slavic word origin of "the kolo" is older than Indo-European and Sanskrit words and means "the wheel-movement," thus inferring to be in a circle and the somatic Slavic folk round dance. Forensic tracing of "Slavic" in language has "ick" word forming as having to do with nature, caused by and being (*Etymology Dictionary* 2023). What the forensics traces as the base of the Slavic languages is the Vedic Sanskrit that stretches for thousands of years and was spoken as late as 300 BCE (Simha 2014). Thus, the somatic matrilineal biological systems, corresponding ecologies, and human societies continue to be at play in the process Bosnian women survivors of war use in the process of healing transgenerational trauma (Anderson 2015b).

There is a great need in the somatic psychological community to understand how cultures across the globe cope with tragic events. For example, the Russian war against Ukraine (2022–) both are of Slavic origins with well over 95 percent Ukrainian women as refugees. A first step is to examine the South Slavic oral memory traditions and how they relate to women's bodies and psyches in the context of war trauma and somatic psychological healing practices, becoming a movement for thriving not surviving (Allen 1996; Campbell 2002; Goldberg et al. 1996; Mertus 2000).

MATERNAL INHERITANCE, LAND, SLAVIC MOIST MOTHER EARTH

I knew in order to narrow down the effects of war trauma on female oral memory traditions, is the focus on the maternal inheritance held within the two specific groups of women from Bosnia-Herzegovina. The striking element found in the first group of Muslim women war crime survivors from Ahmica-Vitez is their rural village where war crimes were committed by the Croatian military upon a Muslim enclave on April 16, 1993 (United Nations 2001). The second group of women war survivors live just two kilometers away in Novi Travnik, a town that once housed a small munitions factory that operated before the war but now is in an entirely different manufacturing field on a socioeconomic precipice. What is outstanding in both of these communities is that they continue to adhere to distinct prewar boundaries dividing the Croatian and Muslim populations. The reason in noting the distinct prewar boundaries are explained with Eastern Bosnian Hercegovina, which are Serbs and Muslim, not Croatians and Muslim populations.

The habitats and environmental factors represented in distinct prewar boundaries andethnic divides presents the geomorphological treacherous sites during war. Added to that is the political strife and corruption in the government, where women are few and often face horrific sexual harassment and attacks if in the legislative body (Simon 2022).

In terms of environmental factors take the example of Perucia. Located in Republic Srpska, eastern Bosnia and Herzegovina, it is one of the last primeval forests reported to be 20,000 years old and is filled with three-hundred-year-old trees (Nevres 2021). With this prime richness of nature, the environmental backdrop is within one of the few primeval forests left in Europe, and along with other resources, continues to be coveted by other countries and greedy corporations. The aftermath of World War I and World War II resulted in many landmines and other buried ordnance in the territory. The Balkan War legacy is a million landmines left in the earth—mostly in Bosnia Hercegovina—adding to the transgenerational trauma.

The interconnection between the life experiences and narratives of South Slavic Muslim women survivors of war crimes and the land reflects a deep relationship between human sociability and the environment (Anderson 2015a). The land holds cultural, historical, and spiritual significance for many communities, including the South Slavic Muslim population.

The land serves as a repository of collective memory, carrying the stories, traditions, and identities of the people who inhabit it. For South Slavic Muslim women survivors of war crimes, the land holds a profound meaning as a tangible link to their heritage and ancestral connections. It provides a sense of belonging, rootedness, and continuity amid the disruptions caused by war and conflict.

I find that the South Slavic Muslim women war crimes survivors' life experiences and women's war crimes narratives containing human sociability behavioral attributes are heavily intertwined with the land (Anderson 2015a). Slavic Moist Mother Earth prehistoric practices evolved into present generations through the use of South Slavic cultural practices and corresponding oral memory traditions (Hubbs 1993). Slavic oral memory traditions are epigenetic and according to the women war survivors are the body—we are all flesh—of deep knowledge excavating down to the roots of problems and obstacles.

The land can be a source of solace, healing, and resilience. Immersion in natural environments and engagement with the land have been shown to have therapeutic effects on individuals who have experienced trauma. Being in nature, connecting with the land, and participating in activities tied to the environment can promote well-being, reduce stress, and foster a sense of connection to something greater than oneself.

Furthermore, the land can serve as a symbolic space for reclaiming agency, asserting cultural identity, and challenging the erasure of women's war crimes narratives. By reaffirming their ties to the land and sharing their stories within the context of their geographic and cultural heritage, South Slavic Muslim women war crimes survivors can assert their presence and move past resilience into thriving, and make contributions to the collective memory.

It is important to recognize the multifaceted relationship between South Slavic Muslim women's experiences, their war crimes narratives, and the land. This interconnectedness highlights the significance of the environment in shaping individual and collective identities, providing a platform for healing, and reaffirming cultural and herstorical/historical legacies.

SOMATIC INFORMED TRAUMA, CULTURE

My inquiry addresses fundamental issues and is poised on Interdisciplinary fields of science, such as cultural psychology, informed trauma, neuroscience, and polyvagal theory approaches. Since the autonomic nervous system responses are in the body-somatic movements and signals from the environment, it is important to note that this study takes place from 1999 to present day—over two decades in Bosnia and Hercegovina middle canton region, in the aftermath of the Balkan War the Russian war on Ukraine.

The Ahmica-Vitez women war crimes survivors are agrarian; they are farmers in a rural village where war crimes were committed by the Croatian military (United Nations 2001). It was mostly the grandmothers, stari babas

(Bosnian Muslim), who were tending to the land and cows when the genocide was committed. The trauma of hearing and witnessing the death screams of infant grandchildren, children, and relatives and seeing their bodies is a never-forgotten wound, according to one Ahmica-Vitez grandmother, and she would not want any grandmother to face such a loss.

Vitez has a large Croatian-owned shopping center and car dealerships on the main road that are mostly owned and operated by Croatians. Since Ahmica-Vitez, like most South Slavic towns, villages are named after families living there for generations. Ahmica is a Muslim family name while Vitez is more or less a Croatian namesake. On the outskirts of the Ahmica-Vitez town, the Muslim farming enclave is located directly across one main road from the Croatian (Catholic) suburb. Many of the sessions were scheduled between growing seasons and harvesting the land.

The second group of women lived just two kilometers away in Novi Travnik, a village that once housed a small munitions factory that operated before the war and is known as an alpine town surrounded by mountains. Since geomorphically, Novi Travnik is a town surrounded by the towering Vrancia (Serbo-Croatian for brown) Mountains, Croatian snipers during the Balkan War incurred dramatic loss of Muslim lives through shooting at the Muslim enclave, and then as a result starvation took place.

Then, there are the million or more landmines embedded in the land and in the mountains surrounding Novi Travnik that continue to terrorize the population. According to journalist Mladen Lakic (2019), "since 1996, when the demining process started in Bosnia and Herzegovina after the war, a total of fifty-five Bosnian deminers and six hundred and seventy-three civilians have been killed by exploding ordnance."

What both groups had in common was a single road in Ahmica-Vitez and also in Novi Travnik, a street that divided the Muslims and Croatians. Another common factor is that the women in these communities survived a legacy of a century of war and holocaust (that is, World War I, World War II, and the Balkan War). While providing cross-cultural and engendered trauma treatment and training, I discovered that neither the women's experiences with war nor their embodied experiences—ranging from physical abuse and rape camps to mass murders of family members—have been clearly identified in order to attempt to improve their lives (Christie and Pim 2012; Mertus 2000; Stiglmayer 1993; Totten 2009). The dehumanizing neglect endured by the two populations of women warrants somatic psychological research, "on inquiring into issues common to anyone working in this field: to think out actual human problems" (Johnson and Grand 1998, 15).

The two groups of Bosnian women have participated and continue to participate in a series of trauma treatment sessions, seminars, and cultural events with me since 2000, during which time somatic psychological practices were incorporated into the traditional kolo dances and/or circles to heal war trauma experienced by the women. A great amount of data was obtained during the period, with extensive field notes, training materials, and cultural traditions captured by the author.

The rich data cycles through evaluation, both descriptively and quantitatively, identifying common themes of coping and of healing that are experienced by the women. A deep understanding of the women's experiences is necessary to accurately assess the effects of the treatment methods. The informed trauma treatment approach integrates knowledge and insights from various sources, including direct experiences with survivors, research findings, and theoretical frameworks. This multidimensional inclusive perspective allows for a deeper exploration of the impacts of kolo, a traditional South Slavic dance and healing practice, on trauma treatment.

The kolo-informed trauma treatment approach, which incorporates a comprehensive understanding of the women's experiences, allows for a unique and valuable perspective within the healing community: it's about learning from one another since the women war survivors are the experts (Anderson 2015a). By integrating their experiences and insights, the treatment approach becomes more effective and tailored to the specific needs of the women and thus of the entire local community (Anderson 2015a, Mertus 2000).

To gain a comprehensive assessment and understanding of the effects of kolo (referring to a specific healing practice or intervention) on the psychological treatment of trauma, it is important to combine these experiential accounts with a thorough review of relevant literature regarding somatic psychological processes in relation to women and trauma. By incorporating both experiential knowledge and existing research, a more nuanced and comprehensive understanding of the therapeutic effects of kolo continues to be achieved.

This all-inclusive approach, combining lived experiences, the creation of the ability to thrive rather than simply survive patriarchal cults, and evaluative data analysis, contributes to a deeper understanding of the impacts of kolo on trauma treatment and provides valuable insights for the movement from survival to thriving and thus healing community.

The current and lived experiences of the South Slavic women who have survived war provide unique and personal insights into the effects of kolo on trauma treatment. The firsthand accounts of individuals who have undergone the treatment can shed light on their subjective experiences, challenges, and transformative processes. These experiences are invaluable in capturing the nuances and intricacies of the healing journey.

Data analysis of South Slavic women who have survived war crimes and war allows for a systematic examination of patterns, themes, and outcomes that emerge from a collection of data. By analyzing the data, researchers can identify commonalities, trends, and variations in the experiences of individuals who have engaged in kolo as a form of trauma treatment. This analytical approach provides a rigorous and objective and subjective understanding of the impacts of kolo and helps to identify factors that contribute to its effectiveness.

Indeed, a comprehensive appraisal is essential for contextualizing the findings of the impacts of kolo on trauma treatment within the existing body of knowledge and research. By conducting a thorough review of relevant research as it pertains to women who have survived war crimes and war and how they heal, researchers and practitioners can identify knowledge gaps.

By integrating lived experiences, data analysis, and literature review, the understanding of the impacts of kolo on trauma treatment is enriched and refined. This inclusive approach ensures that the findings are supported by a robust evidence base, enhancing the validity, applicability, and relevance of the research. Ultimately, it provides valuable insights and guidance for the healing community, helping inform and improve trauma treatment practices.

The informed trauma process is to learn from the women survivors of war crimes and of war about their capacity to heal a century's worth of transgenerational trauma. Therefore, to analyze, interpret, and describe the healing effects of the kolo as related to trauma and psychological treatment is an archaeology of memory found in the culture and in the women's collective.

The data on South Slavic oral memory traditions addresses a vacuum in the treatment of transgenerational trauma, war crimes, and the aftermath of trauma. Current and past research neglects trauma impacts and, specifically, how female oral memory traditions embedded in somatic psychological practices affect female war survivors as viable tools for treating man-made trauma (Anderson 2015a Mertus 2000).

South Slavic women have endured generations of war stress, which continues to affect their sharing of oral memory traditions, the methods of sharing information from one generation to the next (Mertus 2000; Jablonka and Raz 2009). The dehumanizing neglect endured by the two populations of women warrants somatic psychological research to better understand how bodily movements during kolo practices affect emotional healing. However, there is a lack of research pertaining to how the female body and mind respond to the impact of trauma (Fisher and Ogden 2009). There is also a lack of research pertaining to South Slavic culture and corresponding oral memory traditions and the impact of trauma on these survivors (Anderson 2015b; Mertus 2000; Fisher and Ogden 2009).

CULTURE, HOMEOSTATIC HEALING

In turn, women war survivors, who include my mother, defined culture as the homeostatic healing skill space and as a place visible to them and to all females (Anderson 2015a). Therefore, culture is a conglomerate of adaptive transgenerational transformational change and of social cohesion—communal collectives that have evolved to formulate a natural healing culture (Rubin 1995; Anderson 2015b).

Knowing the definitive difference of what encompasses culture is critical. First, culture is not transgenerational trauma, it is maternal epigenetic inheritance for thriving. While culture is epigenetic-transgenerational, the difference is that culture is epigenetic in nature, and it moves toward thriving. At the same time, culture is vulnerable to survival mechanisms (Perez and Lehner 2019; Porges 2011). Culture is an epigenetic incredibly heritable adaptive movement rather than a resilience movement that is embedded in transgenerational survival mechanisms (Porges 2007). Culture contains skills for discoveries of emergence (Wheeler 2006b, 90). Knowing when to apply survival mechanisms and when to flourish is essentially culture that is neurobiologically wired to the environment and to the human body and mind (Damasio 2018; Laney and Bernstein 2020).

Whereas much of clinical trauma and psychology center on resiliency and stress management to cope, resiliency is not a thriving skill set; it is a survival mechanism (Kauffman 2016; Porges 2011). Victims import the message from resiliency psychological efforts that they will need to survive endless transgenerational trauma (Anderson 2012b; Sarkissian and Sharkey 2021). Therefore, resiliency is a life-or-death skill in a world of violence conflicting with the movement from survival to thriving. Flourishing culture in situations of life and death is a matter of knowing when to respond with survival mechanisms and when to employ thriving.

Women war crimes and war survivors felt great conflict with the push to be resilient in the aftermath of the Balkan War. Their reasoning is poised upon healing transgenerational trauma that encompasses prizing both thriving and survival mechanisms. Often remarking how those moments are instructive, a decision point to ask themselves was, "do I need to survive right now or to thrive?" This remains a critical juncture constructed by a culturally specific perspective (Bahtijaragic and Pim 2015).

Therefore, according to the women's survival mechanisms, a neurobiological memory consolidation process, of which resiliency is a part, is only to be employed when needed, not as a remedy to deal with trauma impacts (Kida 2014). The women war survivors said that engaging resiliency was too tiring and mostly exhaustingly divisive (KSW 2000–2022). What becomes apparent is that conflict and violence are accompanied by prejudice, propagating an environment of constant survival readiness. According to social psychologist Muzafer Sherif and his colleagues, in the 1940s and 1950s, researched groups of boys at summer camp with a rival group reported that "when two groups have conflicting aims . . . their members will become hostile to each other even though the groups are composed of normal well-adjusted individuals" (Hopper 2019).

What occurs is the obfuscation of determining when to apply survival mechanisms, and it highlighted when there is a scarcity of resources (Cui et al. 2022). There is the neurobiological empathy mechanism when groups are sharing under scarcity, activating several brain regions "within the mentalizing brain network, but the modulatory effect decreased as a function of cognitive empathy" (Cui et al. 2022).

Interestingly, the women survivors of war crimes and war spoke of sharing a single spoon during the Balkan War and of a collective kolo sharing of resources—the neurobiological empathy mechanisms instead of conflict when facing scarcity (Anderson 2015a; KSW 2000–2022). The resurgence and use of South Slavic maternal oral memory traditions of empathy and of sharing during scarcity of resources, during the Balkan War and in the aftermath, created an adaptive culture.

Survival mechanisms are closely related to fear, which blocks the capacity to decide if the situation requires survival or thriving (Kida 2014; Bentz et al. 2013). As a result, resiliency's coping strategies are neurophysical and autonomic, like breathing to the mind and body, and have many remaining within the physiology of fear, the survival mechanism of fright/flight (Kauffman 2016; Porges 2011).

Transgenerational trauma normalizes behavioral responses rooted in the need to survive violence. Thus, it has perpetuated the patriarchal cult of violence and ongoing femicide for generations (Anderson 2015b; Damasio 2018; Goueffic 2016). Paramount for healing are inquiries about why women's transgenerational trauma is invisible and why it is labeled as a "culture" of violence against women instead of a patriarchal state of violence against primarily women (Zajicek and Calasanti 1998). It is critical to understand women's trauma impacts in past generations into future generations to create an adaptive fluid culture opposed to the physiology of fear and survival mechanisms (Goettner-Abendroth 2012; Eisler 1987).

WOMEN'S TRANSGENERATIONAL TRAUMA AND FEMALE BIOLOGY

Women's transgenerational trauma begins with female biology since the body and mind are intertwined and, under the patriarchy, tightly controlled and thus targeted in violence and wars (Fehr 2011; Goueffic 2016; Wheeler 2006b). Stephen W. Porges's (2011) polyvagal theory emphasizes the functional difference between vagal fibers in the brain stem and found that there are two types of pathways having different embryological origins that "promote different response strategies and provide the neurophysiological justification for new definitions and explanations of stress, distress and distress vulnerability" (91).

The use of patriarchal institutionalizing language with the power to name, to label women as invisible, is femicide since it ignores female biology and vulnerability to distress. Louise Goueffic (2016) notes "patriarchy's evil intent to commit femicide by language. Since language expresses culture, it is cultural femicide." Biology severely diminishes and incessantly thwarts women's ability to operate within social and adaptive culture.

Only recently have genetic sciences revealed what is invisible in the male data sciences, that mitochondrial DNA (mtDNA) is exclusively female—the mothers' egg is matrilineal in nature. However, the sciences label mtDNA matrilineal as maternal inheritance instead of sourcing maternal inheritance as the origin of culture for transmission of flourishing behaviors (Greiner et al. 2015). In Eva Jablonka and Marion J. Lamb's (2005) book, *Evolution in Four Dimensions: Genetic, Epigenetic, Behavioral and Symbolic Variation in the History of Life*, the authors describe maternal inheritance and culture through symbols and genetic information. To be transgenerational and epigenetic, it "has to be used before it is transmitted or acquired by behavioral means. It is easy to see this if you think about how a song or dance is transmitted to others" (Jablonka and Lamb 2005, 202).

For example, when South Slavic women survivors of war crimes and war are in a circle (kolo) or dancing the kolo, they understand they are in a movement and/or dancing in the ancestors' footsteps and adding in their current generations' life experiences.

Culture begins with a maternal somatic-biological felt state to mind/body experiences that produces healing processes and reoccurring cultural interventions into future generations (Damasio 2018; Jablonka and Lamb 2005, 29). Antonio Damasio (2018) posits that "the crucial biological phenomena—feelings and intellect within cultural minds—are only one part of the story. . . at the same time, we need to recognize that the adaptations and faculties used by cultural minds were the result of natural selection and genetic transmission" (29).

But, with the rarity of research into transgenerational trauma-inclusion that focuses on female biology, the question arises about what to do with a study by Mark Schoofs, the geneticist who determined that "every person on Earth in our day can trace their lineage back to a common female ancestor and names her Mitochondrial Eve" (qtd in Asala 2020). Certainly, it places women as originators and creators of culture, a crucial medium from which to heal transgenerational trauma (Anderson 2015a).

Since genetic tools synchronize life, a homeostasis, Damasio (2018) promotes "a working hypothesis on the relations between feelings and culture. Feelings as deputies of homeostasis are the catalysts for response that began human cultures" (26). The Bosnian women war survivors understand and continue to endure femicide that culture addresses as urgent crises of life-and-death situations, and demand healing the transgenerational trauma through their culture, moving from survival to thriving.

CONCLUSION

When trauma is transgenerationally incited by violence, often the violence that accompanies war, survival does not move toward thriving or flourishing. But transformational change is where culture could provide the movement to flourishing (Green et al. 203). Eva Jablonka and Marian J. Lamb (2005) cite intentional learning, not just at the local culture level, but also at the human sociability level that is inclusive of women as creators of culture and requires that it must be culturally acquired (204). Jablonka and Lamb define culture as "the system of socially transmitted patterns of behavior, preferences, and products of animal activities that characterize a group of social animals" (205).

It was my mother's invisibility and silence, and her unending need to survive her internment at a former Yugoslav World War II Jasenovac concentration camp, plus over two decades of informed trauma care with South Slavic women war crimes and war survivors, that propelled my intensive search for healing practices. These practices are found in their South Slavic culture (Anderson 2015a). Since culture moves from survival to flourishing mechanisms, creating the corresponding oral memory traditions, a ritual memory science, neurobiologically is aligned to human sociality (Damasio 2018). But, the South Slavic and Slavic cultures, which houses millennia-old prevention tools, are often discounted and overlooked by the sciences (Ilieva and Shturbanova 1997).

Wendy Wheeler (2006b), in her book *The Whole Creature: Complexity, Biosemiotics and the Evolution of Culture*, points to "an exclusive focus on reductionism and the mechanistic metaphor introduced by seventeenth-century European science . . . it is life and social sciences that have suffered most from this kind of approach" (29). However, these Slavic cultural methods paved an insight into the only possible prevention of infectious holocaustic femicide transgenerational trauma, which is excluded in the sciences and humanitarian agencies (Anderson 2015a; Perez 2021).

All these international and national experiences, especially those that are intangible, if not invisible, prompted me to research the most culturally engendered somatic and polyvagal trauma treatments for the advancement of a framework to overcome the knowledge gap (Porges 2011).

Chapter 2

Invisible

The informed trauma of women war crimes and war survivors revealed an important discovery, a problem statement: It is very apparent that there continues to be very little data and narratives on the *impact of women's trauma.* The stark reality that the scientific categories of human lethal violence are a consensus of male data bias (patriarchal) serves to highlight the role that transgenerational men play as predators; lethal violence "is overwhelmingly a male occupation" (Perez 2021, 2; Goueffic 2016).

You can find entire libraries of women's war crimes and war traumas in the roles of victims or of the deceased. Two elements that are invisible are the impact that this trauma has on women and how women are creators of culture that heals transgenerational trauma. The focus is on the transgenerational nature of trauma, due to its being epigenetic, shaping and influencing of our DNA through life experiences manifested via female biology. An ecosphere of human sociality houses culture (Wheeler 2006b; Damasio 2018).

Therefore, the rarity of studies and information on South Slavic women survivors of war crimes and war whose transgenerational trauma spans a century of wars—World War I, World War II, and the Balkan War—is not acknowledged and is invisible in the sciences, let alone in the media (Goueffic 2016; Mertus 2000). Instead, it is buried in sanctioned victim roles for women (Green et al. 2003; Perez 2021; Goueffic 2016).

Only recently, the outcry for the inclusion of women in data sciences and in the social sciences has acknowledged the lethal violence women continue to endure. According to Caroline Criado Perez (2021), in her landmark book *Invisible Women: Data Bias in a World Designed for Men* states, "the result of this deeply male-dominated culture is that the male experience, the male perspective, has come to be seen as universal, while the female experience—that of half the global population, after all—is seen as, well, niche" (12).

The niche Perez (2021) writes of is the invisibility of women in the data sciences, and thus in trauma that, when studied, belittle women's trauma and determine her female biology and trauma impacts to be insignificant.

Recently, in the bioarchaeological science investigating trauma and violence paper *reports* only "often associated with social spheres of influence and power connected to daily life. Some forms of ritual violence also have restorative and regenerative aspects that strengthen community identity. Viewed in a biocultural context, evidence of osteological trauma provides rich insights into social relationships and the many ways that violence is embedded within those relationships" (Martin and Harrod 2015). The authors do acknowledge and highlight that females are human to create biocultural context—the human sociability and the importance of daily life. The latter has epigenetic, thus transgenerational, value for healing transgenerational trauma.

Another significant piece of my research revealed that refugees are overwhelmingly women, mostly illiterate and poor globally, with few exceptions (Mertus 2000). To address women's trauma and issues, prompts an urgent need to protect and restore, sustaining the benefits that people derive from healthy adaptive and enabling conditions including knowledge (Global Women's Institute 2017; Taub 2022).

Given the critical importance of healing women's trauma and recognizing women as the major caregivers and resources in wars, it is essential to recognize that the aftermath of war women survivors is not represented as such in the global dataset. Instead, women are captured as indicators in the role of victims, not as a resource (Murthy and Lakshminarayana 2006; Perez 2021). Access to gender- related factors is needed to maintain a strong focus on the local women who are the real experts and creators of culture. Regarding women as a resource and not a target in violence and wars can help to accurately assess the needs of the impacted population. Mainstreaming women occurs in humanitarian efforts and in the sciences at this point (Lafreniere et al. 2019; Mertus 2000).

One attempt to mainstream women as culture makers is the United Nations humanitarian effort for women. The United Nations incorporated the archaic ritual of dance in their Valentine's Day "One Billion Rising" project (Pollack 2013). This was a response to the statistic that over a billion women will experience gender-based violence (Pollack 2013). The One Billion Rising project did not contain the word "women" in the title, but the project attempted to include women as a resource for healing transgenerational trauma. When women are not placed in the peripheral role of victims nor discounted and segregated into women-only projects, the healing of transgenerational trauma begins (Global Women's Institute 2017; Murthy and Lakshminarayana 2006).

Analogies can be drawn across the globe, even in countries that experience war in more covert ways. It is intangible. Their cultural oral memory traditions, if used to heal themselves and stop the transgenerational trauma cycle, encourages the flourishing actions and behaviors needed to prevent another generation of trauma born of violence and wars.

EMBODIED PRACTICES

Both the round dance and being in a circle are the embodied practices that have been carried down through the generations as South Slavic culture and female society. South Slavic culture expresses sociocultural communications that foster embodied expressions in approaches to somatic psychological theory and practice. Those practices are carried into moments as needed, particularly in situations of war and of violence, as in the last century of war in the former Yugoslavia (Christie and Pim 2012).

In review of the archives, the kolo applied practices encompass embodied responses based on the wide range of life experiences of the South Slavic women survivors of war crimes and war. Searching for the healing interventions of the South Slavic women, the participants repeatedly pointed to the embodied responses present in the intangible heritage of the Mesolithic kolo. According to Kerewsky-Halpern, in the Balkan bajalica folk healing tool, the collective wisdom of the past is retained and transmitted orally in present-generation healers through communication (building trust, conversation, and touch) (Kerewsky-Halpern 1985). Stephen Porges (2011). The bajalica treatment is found in social engagement which for Slavic peoples describes the importance for ritual psychomania-conflict of the soul endeavoring for the best quality of life. Additionally, the Balkan bajalica and its Western counterpart, polyvagal theory applications, are concerned with cultural connections and physiological responses for possible behavior modification.

A war survivor and resident of the mother city Travnik, located about eight miles from Novi Travnik, spoke of the hundreds of rape camp victims who were seeking refuge in the well-defended city with Mt. Vlasic as its backbone. She shared the story of how a circle of rape camp victims had a ritual of breaking bread before eating. Afterward, the women stood grasping each other's arms and swayed back and forth in a kolo dance. The most memorable part of the story for the war survivor was the comment of the oldest rape camp survivor, who announced, "Now, I am home."

Somatic synchrony is another embodied Slavic oral memory practice. Kolo-applied somatic practices pull in cultural arts, neuroscience, and somatic psychology via intercultural communication, describing why the intangible heritage of the Mesolithic kolo continues to yield healing effects in the aftermath of the most traumatic situations. The kolo dance and the circle include somatic movements that trigger mirror neurons (as in learning through mimicry) and somatic empathy (Iacoboni 2009). In a compelling interview with a Novi Travnik matriarch in 2002, the war survivor of both World War II and the Balkan War described how the kolo dance involves breath so that all participants were breathing and exhaling in rhythm. The matriarch went on to state more observations of the kolo dance. Field notes revealed her input on the kolo as not only important in its sense of movement, but also in just being in a circle, as a place of synchronized movement. Essentially, she stated that we learn from each other not only with words, but also with the body as a social collective. At one point, she suddenly yawned, and within a minute I had yawned as well. Laughing outright, she noted the synchronized movement, proclaiming it to be contagious because our bodies are in constant communication with one another.

The matriarch reported on the superconscious ability of the kolo. Other superconscious abilities include menstruation and pregnancy, in addition to yawning. As Robert E. Svoboda (1986) (Great Mother worship) remarked, "While all the animals yawn, even fish and reptiles—psychotics or the severely ill rarely do, in whom yawning is often a sign that they are beginning to recover. Do not suppress yawning" (53). Thus, the practice of yawning appears to be in line with our healthy mental states, so it follows that yawning synchronicity may be evoked during healing practices.

Along with the South Slavic matriarch, eight other female survivors of the Balkan War reported in the 2002 focus group that they knew that yawning and bleeding together were steps of synchronization (Knight 1995). According to the respondents, the kolo is synchronicity that leads toward solidarity and is based on their life experiences of raising children and growing food from the "Moist Mother Earth." The South Slavic female war survivors' intimate wisdom of the body's way of learning is similar to that which scientists call the *mirror-neuron system* (Rossi 2002). The mirror-neuron circuitry system "contains a special type of brain cells, or neurons, that become active both when their owner does something, and when he or she senses someone else doing the same thing" (taken from http://www.world-science.net/exclusives/050309_yawnfrm.htm; qtd. Cossu 2012). These neurons are activated upon the conscious imitation of someone else's actions, as in learning. In the case of yawning, the mirror neuron system may become activated subconsciously.

The applied somatic psychology practices found in the kolo have a deep ecological embracement. For example, the matriarchs understood that contagious yawns, as repeating and replicating behaviors, do not begin with the left-brain functions of reason or of logic. Yawning, as a practice, strikes at the core of what is universal from the seat of being: healing practices that represent the ability to have and to be a part of great movements (Christie and Pim 2012). The archived material revealed that the respondents referred to other abilities of synchrony, such as ovarian synchrony, as a result of kolo movements and superconscious abilities (Knight 2002; Kalof 2012).

However, heRobert Hershey et al. (2014) in "Mapping Intergenerational Memories (Part I): Proving the Contemporary Truth of the Indigenous Past," state that there is a limitation on indigenous communities' oral memory traditions (kolo) that label intergenerational memories as not having concrete methods or not being lineal enough for Western theories. This may explain how somatic practices found in diverse cultures and oral memory practices were disregarded or ignored.

WHAT CONTINUES AND WHAT COMES NEXT?

There is no epilogue due the transgenerational trauma and continued exploitation of women who are the main targets of conflict, wars, domestic violence/ nonstate torture and second-class citizenry. The research and trauma response of biodata, forensics, biometric, sociometric, and especially psychometric measurement concentrated on the cultural and social aspects in healing trauma of women survivors of war crimes and war d. The female body and her human mind display the exploitation of human labor but also highlight women's key roles in healing transgenerational trauma.

I developed and applied my kolo-informed trauma program, and as one result I was inducted into the UNESCO Council of Dance scientific and education section in 2020. The women survivors of war crimes and war and I were recognized for the two decades of kolo-informed transgenerational trauma healing through oral memory traditions and research on the Balkan route and pathways.

Qualitative description and qualitative research continue to be accomplished as a core part of the kolo informed trauma program and concurrent Balkan route and pathways research project. Why? Information evolves us. We have consciousness and growth. Fieldwork, interviews, and clinically informed trauma practices with South Slavic Bosnian Balkan War survivors who fled on the Balkan route, and pathways are currently inhabited by the Afghan, African, and Syrian refugees with their unending transgenerational trauma narratives (Anderson, 2015a). They provide more insight into women refugees, transgenerational trauma, and their need for safety and a durable and life-sustaining cultural refugee response from governments and military and humanitarian aid agencies. However, my research and kolo-informed trauma on South Slavic women survivors of war crimes and war is rare and little known.

The current updates have the Slavic Ukrainian women refugees using the Balkan route, which unsurprisingly yields a women's transgenerational trauma narrative since over 90 percent are women with more than half children (UN Women, April 5, 2022, Rapid gender analysis in Ukraine reveals different impacts and needs of women and men). However, as before in World War I, World War II, and the Balkan War, women are on the front lines but not in the headlines and do not predominate in humanitarian aid funding, response, or trauma studies as a focus. The fact that research generalizes from the experiences of men obscures the healing resources and trauma responses unique to women. Media portrays the Ukrainian mothers as the heart of the war, which signals their sacrificial victim role (Vohra 2022).

Given, the Balkan route has a majority of refugees with experience of transgenerational trauma and war crimes which is a cultural oral memory adaptive movement—an embodied circle and dance and the memory of processions. Somatic (body) and tacit knowledge that is not taught. In fact, consciousness erupts with movement (Wheeler 2016). Tacit knowledge and oral memory traditions (a ritual science) create adaptive cultures for healing trauma (Anderson 2015a; Rotramel 2019). The research and interviews with refugees indicate a tacit knowledge resource, a transgenerational trauma survival procession movement, and fleeing violence. With seeking safety, it is to create an adaptative culture (Anderson 2015a; Lehrner and Yehuda 2018).

The South Slavic women survivors of war crimes and war along with the Balkan Route women refugees' tacit knowledge identified four phases guiding my exploration and research include the following: engagement, immersion into the Balkan route and women refugees, highlighting the relationship between women and their social surroundings, their mutual need blocked by obstacles women refugees must navigate through and negotiate, and the needed change required to create an adaptative movement.

While the story of kolo-informed trauma treatment with South Slavic women survivors of war crimes and war story began in Bosnia, the impact of war crimes mostly likely would occur at the site of recent and past genocides with brutal wars that have displaced and traumatized its people in unspeakable ways. All over the world, women, men and children have suffered immeasurably from horrific acts of violence in counties such as Kenya, the Congo, Rwanda, India, Sri Lanka, the Sudan and Uganda. Not only does the violence traumatize those who face it, the trauma remains with its victims wherever they travel and is passed down generation after generation.

LITERACY OF ABUNDANCE

The reality is, nothing has been effective in facing this grossly fecund intergenerational trauma—or finding a way to heal the wounds it causes. Women and children, especially young girls, bear the brunt of much of the violence perpetuated throughout the world. According to author Theodor Winkler

(2005), violence against women is the fourth-leading cause of premature death on the planet, ranking behind only disease, hunger, and war.

"We are confronted with the slaughter of Eve, a systematic gendercide of tragic proportion," wrote Winkler (2005) in his book *Women in an Insecure World*. Unfortunately, many in the international community do not even consider rape a war crime. To explore explored trauma impacts and violence in the kolo-informed trauma treatments with women and children is not done only in their victim roles that often turns them into poster models for humanitarian aid agencies and allies. Yet, despite such media exposure and new rules of law concerning rape as war crimes, the ripple effect of trauma continues, scarring entire communities around the globe.

The Slavic kolo, an ancient round dance and circle tradition tracing beyond Paleolithic origins has been known to South Slavs for generations since it shares the amenities of organized social life based on collaboration and peace before war became a modern reality. The kolo tradition witnesses traumatized women, such as those in Bosnia who have experienced three wars in the past one hundred years. Through the kolo, witnessing enables people to escape the human bondage to intergenerational trauma and the war environment.

An integral part of the kolo, whether dancing the round folk dances or being in a circle, is the concentrated collective ability to bear witness and share one's story. The kolo circle remains within Slavs' consciousness as if it were the only thing from their past that could not be erased.

First, the way in which the women grew to understand that in healing their own trauma, they heal that of all others. The second aspect was their refusal to hover between realms of war and violence. They chose instead to bring an archaic cultural symbolism into the aftermath of war so that the literacy of abundance and peace prevails. The women war crimes and war survivors understood that safety from the patriarchal institutions and political realm was had in their social engagements in the kolo. It is a place and space to share their stories, they are able to author a nonviolent sequel to their lives—and the lives of their children.

The women are empowered by a safe and ancient archeomythologies of Old Europe, a symbolic process that does not offend or provoke the ire of patriarchal religions or governing entities. The process ultimately leads to the painful but necessary bearing witness—communal applications of wisdom, resiliency, only triggered in survival modes and moved into thriving life skills. And by bearing witness among those with whom they share the circle, the women remember that they are empowered to heal their families and communities.

The kolo's universal communal features revokes any outside authority by empowering women to remember they manifest culture and are the healers of their global communities—societies where women and children are not invisible or erased.

Chapter 3

Social Memories

While the field of somatic psychology calls into question the very meaning of *body*, both in theory and practice (Kampe 2010; Nickerson 2022), there exists a gender bias in the development of somatic psychological practices. The female body is of particular interest to somatic psychology (McCarthy 2004). However, somatic psychological research has focused on male embodiment based on the assumption that men's and women's bodies are similar, if not strictly because of an abundance of male researchers who may envision the generic human as male (Perez 2021).

On the contrary, female biological processes have the capacity to create social memories by forging culture through daily life, pregnancies, child-rearing, domestic life, and relationships, which may represent the earliest known origins of somatic psychology, polyvagal treatments, and cultural psychology (Porges 2011; Damasio 2018; Knight 2002; Kalof 2012).

Culture is defined as the vehicle for collective memories with the capacity to organize shared cultural knowledge into successive generations (Confino 1997). The shared cultural knowledge for South Slavic peoples is known as *oral memory traditions*, an intangible heritage with varying interrelations among vastly differing memories that capture the epigenetic habits that effect modalities of change and recognize patterns and disruptions (Damasio 2018, Anderson 2015b).

Culture and collective memories are especially significant for South Slavic female Muslim war crimes and war survivors due to genocide and femicide memories from World War I, World War II, and the Balkan War (Hunt 1989; Wilson 1996). The result is the oral memory traditions' adaptive outcomes of expectations, social engagement, and bonding.

Looking at the expectations of oral memory traditions, they are about the information and messages from the environment we live in so as to elevate growth—evolving pathways to thrive and to know when to survive (Anderson 2015b). Participants in the social engagements found in the kolos—either to be in a circle or folk round dance—report being in relationships with all life. And the bonding that is formed in the perinatal, natal, and child-rearing periods is made possible to be expressed in communal collectives (Anderson 2021, 19).

Despite the close ties between culture and somatic psychology, scientific research has failed to seriously consider the relationship between the oral memory traditions of South Slavic women and somatic psychological practices. Regarding the rarity of women's transgenerational trauma consequences and their cultural memory and oral memory practices in data and in the cultural and psychological to neuroscience fields directed the research to look at what is intangible—invisible.

In fact, cultural memory created by symbolic inheritance, embodied in text, rites, movements of the body, and feelings, are mnemonic epigenetic instigators so the intangible memory can be evoked, recalled, and regenerated throughout generations (Meckien 2013). Communicative memory is limited only to a recent past event, evoking personal and autobiographic memories, and lasting perhaps three to four generations (Meckien 2013; Rose 2006). According to Jan Assmann and Aleida Assmann, professors define cultural memory as durable (lasting through the ages) and symbolic inheritance that transmit everyday life through orality and intangible cultural memory (Meckien 2013).

Eric Kandel is the leading memory neuroscientist for his research underlying long-term memory and simple reflexes and learned associations (Rose 2006). Kandel received the Nobel Prize in Physiology for his research on the biology of memory showing how learning—what I call intensified learning—produces changes in behaviors by modifying connections between nerve cells and not by altering the basic brain circuitry (Kandel 2023).

Kandel's memory research is not by coincidence. What Kandel shares with the South Slavic Women War Crimes and War survivors is World War II and the Jewish Holocaust (Rose 2006). Kandel's life experiences and his escape to the United States becoming an immigrant who announced himself to be Hitler's first victim makes his research more invaluable to the South Slavic women survivors of war crimes and war.

However, in the past decade more research and data emerged the Ukraine war (2022) where over 90 percent of the refugees are women (Taub 2002).

TACIT KNOWLEDGE

Given the Balkan War (1991–1994) and the Ukrainian War (2022) the field in common is the Slavic culture threaded with matrilineal inheritance thus tacit knowledge revealed in the oral memory traditions (Anderson 2015b; Hubbs 1993;Goettner-Abendroth 2013; Wheeler 2006b). Slavic culture and corresponding oral memory traditions have tacit knowledge—a knowing without being taught since the knowledge is acquired from each person's life experience that is intangible, intuitive. Tacit knowledge is difficult to express through language or images since each person's experiences are a personal knowledge from lived experiences (Wheeler 2006b).

Tacit knowledge essentially is cellular memory (Wheeler 2006b). Our cellular memory, like tacit knowledge, is "human knowledge by starting from the fact we can know more than we can tell" (Polanyi 1966, 4). Statements, usually from women "I know this," face onslaught from male-dominated sciences and dualistic patriarchal either-or demands. Reductionism, narrowed down to the smallest detail, obscures the essence of the female biology found in the mitochondria dynamics (Perez 2021; Pert 1999).

However, in my clinical trauma interactions with the Bosnian women survivors of war crimes and war, I immediately understood the cultural and oral memory transgenerational memory describing the nature of agency—that something can be acted upon—movement, in human consciousness or unconsciousness is evident in human female biological systems.

Women often complain about the fact that cellular learning intelligence—and therefore, their reality—is absent from the sciences. Countless variations of "I know this" from the Bosnian women war crimes and war survivors is epigenetics' cellular memory, which I call tacit knowledge. The women survivors of war crimes and war are pointing to the dissonance, the "failure to pay attention to the ways in which our conceptual knowledge is the product of a disembodied mind" (Wheeler 2006b, 61). Cellular learning intelligence is absent from the sciences and their enworlded realities in life, and that the women say, I know there is no science on this, but this is what I know/intuitively I feel is right-embodied.

The women survivors of war crimes and war with their tacit knowledge, enworlded realities are as a result the academics, the professionals of collective memory, transgenerational trauma memories. At this point, the women war survivors move toward flourishing and do not remain stuck in survival mechanisms (Anderson 2015a).

The sciences and reductive paradigm are explicit knowledge, which is easily codified, written to be shared in journals and books (Wheeler 2006b). At the same time tacit knowledge is intangible; therefore, it is dismissed in the sciences since it highlights the absence of flesh-and-blood narratives, embodied and indwelling (Polanyi 1966). What occurs with culture and oral memory traditions in its absence from the sciences is deemed as not logical and certainly without scientific proof. Richard Brock (2017) argues that while tacit knowledge is inexpressible knowledge and thought "unlikely to be of great importance to teaching and learning science" (133) he thinks the reverse is true. According to Brock, the presence of tacit knowledge and intuitions reflect inexpressible knowledge.

Poring through thousands of studies and quite a few books, it was within UNESCO that the intangible aspects of tacit knowledge were recognized and UNESCO agrees with Brock (2017) on its importance.

> Oral traditions and expressions are used to pass on knowledge, cultural and social values, and collective memory. They play a crucial part in keeping cultures alive. Some types of oral expression are common and can be used by entire communities, while others are limited to particular social groups, only men or women, perhaps, or only the elderly. In many societies, performing oral traditions is a highly specialized occupation, and the community holds professional performers in the highest regard as guardians of collective memory. (UNESCO 2023)

Despite the fact that the South Slavic women war survivors most are without academic background, and a few are illiterate, the women have skillful healing of transgenerational trauma garnered from a century of wars to employ a human sociability toward flourishing (Anderson 2015a; 2015b).

My mother's untold story: a survivor of a World War II concentration camp at Jasenovac gave birth to four daughters and one son in the roles of an invisible female refugee and immigrant (Anderson 2015; Remembrance.org 2022). My mother's invisible status continues to be lived out among women refugees and immigrants in modern-day warfare and violence against women. Despite the research of women's trauma impact on her female biological body and mind is rare when held within the male-biased data science and in the field of psychology for healing trauma, I encountered in my informed trauma an emergence of a new stratum (Perez 2021; Polanyi 1966).

That new stratum I encountered with my mother's silence, her untold story of the World War II Jasenovac concentration camp. Work with women survivors of war was my grasping for a skilled way of healing transgenerational trauma through culture and oral memory traditions.

PAINFUL LEGACIES TO ADAPTIVE EPIGENETIC CHANGES

When such trauma is transmitted from one generation chronically to the next generation, a painful legacy is manifested. However, what I learned from my informed trauma clinical treatment from the South Slavic Muslim women survivors of war crimes and war, it is not to be conflated with culture (Anderson 2012b).

In turn, women survivors, to include my mother, defined homeostasis as a visible place to them and all females,matrilineally (Anderson 2015a; Damasio 2018). This is how culture is a conglomerate of adaptive, epigenetic transgenerational transformational change. One of the homeostasis regulation outcomes is the social cohesion-communal collectives' evolving to formulate a natural healing culture—human flourishing (Rubin 1995; Anderson 2015b; Damasio 2018).

Knowing the definitive difference of what encompasses culture is critical. The reminder is that culture is not transgenerational trauma. Culture is an epigenetic incredibly adaptive movement rather than a ceaseless resilience campaign due to embedded transgenerational survival mechanisms (Green et al. 2003). Culture contains skills for discoveries for emergence (Wheeler 2006b, 90). Knowing when to apply survival mechanisms and when to flourish is essentially culture that is neurobiologically wired to the environment and the human body and mind (Damasio 2018).

Whereas much of clinical trauma and psychology center on resiliency and stress management to cope, resiliency is not a thriving skill set (Kauffman 2016). Thus, transgenerational trauma victims import the message that they will need to survive endlessly transgenerationally for thousands of generations (Anderson 2012b; Sarkissian and Sharkey. 2021). Since resiliency is a life-or-death skill in a world of violence, it often forgoes the movement from survival to thriving, human flourishing (Anderson 2015b; Bentz et al. 2013).

Since survival mechanisms are a fight-or-flight autonomic response and not a neurobiologically sociability memory consolidation process, those survival skills are not to be thrown away (Kida 2014; Cowan et al. 2021). Survival readiness is only to be applied when acutely determined and imperatively required. But, discerning when to move from survival to thriving is almost impossible to do in a patriarchy with numerous wars, violence, and pandemics entrenched in fear, terror fright/flight responses (Eisler 1987; Goettner-Abendroth 2012; Mira et al. 2021).

The latter therein lies the much-needed healing of transgenerational trauma: foster cultural relativism and advocacy stressing the existence of matrilineal processes found in oral memory traditions and women's voices which are voices for change with such cultures themselves (Mertus 2000, 116). In considering both groups, South Slavic women survivors of war crimes and war living in two different towns, despite the lack of mental health and humanitarian programmatic male-ocused policies, were able to be a focal point with the explicit women's role perspectives delimiting the drawbacks and obstacles besetting them in the aftermath of war (Anderson 2015a).

An example of this with the Bosnian war survivors (Novi Travnik) was the marching for garbage pickup in 2001. The huge metal trash containers were spontaneously combusting, bursting into flames often sounding like bullets flying and mortar attacks. The startle reflex with the war survivors and their families was exhibited throughout all. I left to return to the United States when the leader of Kolo Sumejja (Novi Travnik) informed me that she and the women marched for trash pickup services banging pots and pans down the streets (archive Kolo Sumejja Women [KSW] War Crimes and War Survivors 2000–2022).

Eerily, the garbage pickup was done while the women were still marching. The banging pots and pans symbolized their voices of change and their oral memory traditions and domestic life of cooking, their self-sustaining gardens to underline their threat to the men in power, that their dinners will no longer be served.

INSTITUTIONALIZED VIOLENCE AS NORMAL LIFE

Violence against women is normalized under the five-thousand-year reign of the patriarchy and is aptly summarized by author Maria Mies (Mies 1998; Baring and Cashford 1991). Mies (1998) writes, "the battle is not between particular groups within and men and between women and men. Most men and women try to avoid it because they fear that if they allow themselves to become aware of the true nature of man-woman relationship in our societies, the last island of peace, of harmony in the cold brutal work of money-making, power games and greed will be destroyed" (6). With this study of South Slavic women survivors of war crimes and war, the century of wars gives a modern insight into the existence of a patriarchal order through thousands of years—messaging ceaseless violence (Concept Daily 2021; Goettner-Abendroth 2012).

Examples of the continuing institutionalized patriarchal patterns of violence are shown during the Balkan War and in the aftermath. In the presence of black markets and mafia organizations, corruption is the order of business took hold of the economy and greed took hold of governing entities (BBC 2016). Domestic violence/nonstate torture escalated with the unemployment of men loitering in the streets, many of whom dealing with drug and alcohol substance abuse (Kiggins 2021).

In the beginning of my sessions with the Bosnian women survivors of war crimes and war, I asked the women if they say no to their husband's demands that were not the moist mother earth culture but are the entrenched patriarchal cult violence. This was in response to the domestic violence/nonstate torture for the survivors had many women repeating "the war will never end" (KSW 2000–2022).

Comments from the women in their gossip centered on hearing the yelling and the beatings of one woman who did not clean the house properly and another not having dinner on the table for their husbands. What was being encountered was the war entrained the men's instinct to kill, male entitlement to be in control and have power over women.

Returning to Novi Travnik, months later, I was told of that two women who were killed—who said no and did not clean the home properly or have dinner ready. In that session my decision was to halt the informed trauma treatments feeling the deaths of the women was due to the trauma-informed sessions about saying no (KSW 2000–2022).

At that moment, the eldest of the survivors' groups stood up and admonished me. She informed me that I was arrogant to think I had that much power and that it is her work, her sisterhood that needed to create a culture where women are kept safe, honored, and respected. At that moment the narratives of the study's women survivors of war crimes and war tracked women's empowerment to create culture at the local level—from the bottom up—and evidence for rituals of closure.

Hence the importance of older matriarchs as important repositories of healing transgenerational knowledge involved in the study (Anderson 2015b). Additionally, this explains why long-term memory can lead directly to the movement of survival to thriving.

The South Slavic matriarchs in the study navigate what biologists call a "fission-fusion" dynamic. In this arrangement, a core kolo, circle network—matriarchs encounter hundreds of other women during and after the war facing domestic violence/nonstate torture, institutionalized violence against women events (fusion). Through meeting with various communities outside their locale, women war survivors would later return to their local kolo sisterhood (fission) with what was learned.

What resonated an uncannily familiar Slavic transgenerational oral memory rites is the intensified learning to historical—herstories are "interpreted of the more distant past to serve the needs and interests of their present lives" (Van Dyke and Alcock 2003, 1). Digging deeper is how their human sociability is a fusion/fission process that also occurs at the core biological cellular mitochondrial level.

The matrilineal mitochondria-female biology is the major hub to convert energy. The same holds true for in the Bosnian women war crimes and war survivors' empowerment to create a hub, a culture—a human sociability networking (Y. J. Liu et al. 2020). As such, the Bosnian women war crimes and war survivors were operating in a highly complex human sociability platform through the Slavic oral memory tradition of the kolo.

The South Slavic narratives of the flesh—stories and diverse forms of information from the Bosnian women war crimes and war survivors akin to the matrilineal mitochondria process—transmits onward transgenerationally either in oral memory traditions or fixed textual accounts (Van Dyke and

Alcock 2003; Anderson 2015b). For instance, the study revealed how crucial it is to have detailed knowledge of family members and close associates, as well as being able to identify strangers and being more cautious when interacting with these unknown individuals who might act aggressively and pose a threat to the family thus their community (Anderson 2014a; 2015a).

Throughout all the dire and direct war and aftermath war patterns of violence, the Bosnian women survivors of war crimes and war maintained a fluid social cohesion through their oral memory rites. An array of activism, marches for women's human rights and outreach to other sisterhood groups of women such as Bosfam's Srebrenica women war crimes survivors where coffee and kolache (baked goods) were served (Niksic 2021). The informed trauma sessions occurred over steaming demitasse cups of coffee or chai not in an office.

There was no office to be had for the women and rare funding for them. But these excursions are the therapeutic offices that seamlessly removed the Bosnian women war crimes and war survivors from their war-blighted town for short periods. The Bosnian women survivors of war crimes and war went to Sarajevo, Fojnica, Zenica, and to the Bosnian Adriatic coast, funded through international individual donations. Many of the women never left the perimeter of their town since the bus fare of barely fifty cents was too costly before the Balkan war and impossibly high in the aftermath of war.

While the women survivors of war and war crimes joked and teased about how could this is be therapy, dramatic changes took place.

The Slavic women's oral memory traditions involving music, songs to bar jokes occurred on the tattered yellow bus. The baked goods and full-course meals of spit-roasted lamb, oral memory bioculinary rituals were carefully packaged for the excursions, becoming a show-and-tell performance on who is the best chef or the best singer or comedian (Anderson 2012a). Prior to the excursions, the women in their towns to that of the bus rides revealed how these women had stopped laughing, their sense of humor and social cohesion was a rarity (Anderson 2015a).

After a few years the Bosnian women survivors of war crimes and war were on the television and radio programs. An LBGQTIA feminist group, a much younger group from Serbia, hosted the Bosnian women at a performance of Eve Ensler's feminist Monologue at an international televised conference honoring them. The Novi Travnik, Kolo Sumejja women's group leader was given the Vagina Warrior award.

While it was very tenuous and outright risky to ride to the border of Serbia and Bosnia Hercegovina since the kolo of Bosnian women survivors of war crimes and war are Muslim, much discussion ensued, with the Bosnian women survivors and Serbian feminist activists to minimize any opportunity for violence. The Serbian feminist activists were aware of the Balkan War transgenerational trauma targeting women, "other" groups, especially the Muslim religion from Croatians (Catholic) and Serbs (Serbian Orthodox) religious sects.

What occurred was a proliferation within the construction of social memory. Social memory is an active social cohesion and ongoing process forming direct connections among all women war survivors and their remembered past. This is shown by the Serbian activist women's group consulting with the women war survivors the decision on who should receive the Eve Ensler's Vagina Warrior award. The women war survivors concluded the Bosnian Muslim women war survivors' matriarch was the only one with a name that was not Islamic, and she received the award (KSW 2000–2022).

The husbands and male relatives were shocked to see the women on the newscasts. Many of the male relatives came to me asking me what I have done. A few remarked they were grateful for the few years of getting to know me first, respected me and these women because they would have killed me outright or would have said no. Most of the male relatives said they thought I was having "just" coffee and cookies with the women. With my silence to their responses, most of the male relatives remarked it wasn't you, it was "our" women.

MATRILINEAL CULTURE—SOCIAL COHESION

However, pockets of matrilineal culture, what Mies (1998) calls islands of peace and harmony—human flourishing were created in the face of patriarchal violence, war crimes, and war. Despite the taboo of speaking their war narratives, let alone having press conferences and outright testimonies through coordinating with all South Slavic women's groups, South Slavic women survivors of war shared their narratives concerning the rape/death camps and the internment of older women; some of the older women are doctors who performed abortions in cases of forced pregnancies (Allen 1996).

Interviews with the South Slavic women survivors of war concerning the rape/death camps discussed how the older women and especially those who were doctors were targeted (KSW 2000–2022). The war survivors pointed to these women as moving through fear as an indication that female biology, body, and mind—a human sociability, matrilineal female collective erupted (Anderson 2015b; Goettner-Abendroth 2012).

Survival mechanisms are closely related to fear (Kida 2014; Bentz et al. 2014). Two questions arise with the Slavic women in the case of at least thirty rape/death camps and the testimony of rape victims numbering between twenty thousand and fifty thousand women in the Balkan War (Allen 1996).

One question arises, why the crimes are not punished? The shockingly slow legal process was quite violent toward the rape victims, leading to fear, if not terror, in the rape survivors. The women war survivors pointed to transgenerational trauma survival mechanisms at play. Most of the South Slavic survivors responded that fear and terror deplete their energy since they are major caregivers to heal the rape victims (KSW 2000–2022). The second-highest response from the womensurvivors was in the lines of asking the following; if the rapes/death camps in World War I, World War II, and the Balkan War, let alone in Africa, Asian Pacific Islanders rapes were not held accountable or reported, why would the Balkan War women rape victims report the rapes and violence now?

The South Slavic women war survivors' matrilineal female collective stated a social cohesion; they know what transpired, and this is the point that we heal together since it is not possible within patriarchal institutions and rule of law (KSW 2000–2022; Anderson 2015a). The South Slavic war survivors strengthened social cohesion in face of fear and terror and when facing violence or living in a war zone that never ends (Anderson 2015a; Mertus 2000). Social cohesion is an element of matrilineal culture and that of oral memory rites conducted in a collective in their locality (Damasio 2018).

The second question concerns the Slavic matrilineal culture, an earth-based religion that is Mesolithic in age: how did the women survivors of war create culture in the aftermath of wars and violence (Marler 1991; Baring and Cashford 1991). According to Damasio, the human nervous system evolved human life and cognitive features, thus "cultures can be fully explained by biological mechanisms" (Damasio 2018, 28). The Slavic prehistoric culture centered on the Moist Mother Earth (Hubbs 1993; Gimbutas 1991), a matrilineal culture that strengthens social cohesion. How did the mostly uneducated South Slavic survivors of war invite these crucial factors?

The factor concerns the women's confidence in their tacit knowledge (Wheeler 2006b). It is within the tacit knowledge the women war survivors, with none holding an academic diploma, fully comprehended their female biological phenomena, their nervous system/polyvagal theory (Porges 2007) to prompt and shape events—life experiences that become a matrilineal cultural phenomenon.

The intangible matrilineal culture-shaping events globally with many women's groups had something to do with the International Yugoslav War Crimes Tribunal finally mandating that the "mass rape and sexual enslavement in in time of war will for the time be regarded as a crime against humanity, a charge second in gravity only to genocide" in 2001 (Osborn 2001).

What is to be learned is that transgenerational trauma normalizes violence, producing survival mechanisms ruling the women's lives globally. Before the Balkan War mass rape and sexual enslavement camps, there had been holocaustic rapes in Asia-Pacific Islanders and Africa but none of which categorically had the mass rapes listed as a war crime (Ravitz 2011; Kashgarian 2021). Perpetuating the cult of violence, ongoing femicide for thousands of generations and continuing to this present moment, the normalized violence and autonomic survival-fright/flight envelops everyone (Anderson 2015b; Damasio 2018; Goueffic 2016).

Therefore, any inquiries on why women's transgenerational trauma is invisible and labeled a culture of violence against women instead of a cult of violence begins with female biology since the body, the nervous system, and mind are intertwined (Fehr 2011; Goueffic 2016; Wheeler 2006b; Porges 2011).

The South Slavic women's responses to the second question, again spoke of social cohesion; our bodies, we are flesh-and-blood sisterhood making room for a safe place for women to bleed, to birth, and to die (KSW 2000–2022). It was Maria Mies (1998) writing of the hostility that feminists face from large sections of the male population—especially those women who were influential stated that being faced with fear, terror, and violence "only reinforced the feelings of sisterhood" (7).

In the Balkan War rape camps, the older women, some of whom were doctors, performed abortions and other medical services becoming leaders for the women while they were interned. The Bosnian women war survivors knew their names and most of the narratives since these women doctors knew their matriarchal role as influencers (KSW 2000–2022). Given that female' bodies and gender examine women's trauma issues, the divide between sociability inclusive of women and patriarchal forces that shape their respective roles, results in their explicit needs are not attended to thus the target in violence and wars—with unique specific rape war experiences (Mertus 2000, 15; Skjelsbæk 2016).

Since the Slavic sisterhood was facing a forced occupation of their wombs, a wall of silence ensued (Omerovic 2021). For instance, the estimates of the numbers of South Slavic women survivors of war crimes rape vary with no accuracy (Skjelsbæk 2016). In interviews with the Bosnian war survivors, I spoke of how I have yet, to meet or know a child of rape during my two decades of clinical trauma treatments (KSW 2000–2022; Omerovic 2021). However, the Bosnian women war survivors had more accuracy of the rape war crimes and kept the origin of the children contained in their sisterhood (S. K. Fisher 2006; Anderson 2015b).

One of the elder Bosnian women survivors of war took me aside in an interview before my return to the United States. The elder commenced a lament raging against the international humanitarian agencies to the US customs concerning visas. In a powerfully influencing narrative she instructed me not ask any South Slavic women when they came to the United States. I was unsure how she knew it was my line of questioning as it was in line with the international humanitarian agencies and US customs.

The realization that the kolo sisterhood (Slavic folk round dance or to be in a circle) extended to me provided the awareness of blaming the rape war victim and not healing transgenerational trauma. The sex and gender perspective in the Slavic oral memory traditions filled with culturally intensified learning accepted the reality of patriarchal control and rule over their wombs. The elder, illiterate, barely got through the second-grade elementary schooling due to World War II, had her tacit knowledge and use of the South Slavic oral memory traditions to give explicit attention to collective trauma women rape war victims endure even with diaspora (KSW 2000–2022).

That information concerned US visas given to South Slavic war and rape war survivors between 1991–1995 because they were only given to the rape victims and their families. Therefore, asking when did the former Yugoslav women come to the states, literally tells the person or institution that she has been raped and offered a special visa. In my interviews with former Yugoslav women stateside when I did inquire the number of years they had lived in the United States, I encountered a distrusting and distressing silence (KSW 2000–2022).

In the end, the Bosnian war survivors in this study war rape experience are a South Slavic and Slavic cultural collective oral memory narrative recognizing the sheer "totality in which war rapes occurred" (Skjelsbæk 2016, 373). Hence, the invisibility of women's war rape and war experiences and narratives data where the number of raped women ranges from twenty thousand to fifty thousand (S. K. Fisher 2006).

Even more perturbing is the data science uncertainty in the estimates of how many children were conceived in war rapes, with an estimate from the Bosnian Ministry of Works and Social Affairs reporting that 35,000 women rape war survivors were impregnated (Skjelsbæk 2016). The male-biased science went on the offensive reporting the statistic that one single act of intercourse resulting in pregnancy ranges from 1 to 4 percent, therefore it would be an impossible 3,500,000 acts of rape that took place in the Balkan War (Skjelsbæk 2016; Perez 2021).

The logic of using the 1 to 4 percent resulting in pregnancy and calculating the number of rapes using the general averages of sexual intercourse conceiving a child is misapplied. Yes, the totality of 3,500,000 intercourse acts is known to be the average of conceiving a child across a vast general population. But what and where is the data concerning the total number of mass rapes conceiving a child in a rape enslavement camp, in an institution such as military to date rape?

The Bosnian women war survivors' sisterhood from healing their collective transgenerational trauma has a female coherent interior field becoming a crucial part of their matriarchal cultural agreement to engage in healing, which is to flourish. Receiving accurate data not just on the Bosnian women rape war survivors but the Bosnian women war survivors developed a depth of integration in face of transgenerational fear and terror (Hubl 2020, 117).

Furthering my argument, the use of matriarchal culture and corresponding oral memory traditions in language is a patriarchal institutionalizing language with the power to name, to label women as invisible—femicide while ignoring female biology. Goueffic states "patriarchy's evil intent to commit femicide by language. Since language expresses culture, it is cultural femicide" (Goueffic 2016). To operate as both a social and female biological being is severely diminished and incessantly thwarted from creating an adaptive and evolving thriving culture in their environment (Anderson 2015b; Cockburn 2013).

A target heavily used during the Balkan War was discussed by the Bosnian war survivors. It encompassed their starvation and the snipers killing them as they fled to markets or the countryside for food (KSW 2000–2022; Anderson 2012a). Cut off from their Moist Earth sustenance, their apartment balconies with pots of vegetables and herbs, and backyards to the town's marketplace, were targeted by snipers and mortar attacks that were ever present in their geosphere of daily life. It resulted in many deaths of women and children (Anderson 2012b).

It's not just the Balkan women survivors of war, it's global especially in conflict, poverty, racism, and war regions. For example, what happens to her in the Balkan War attacks will happen to everyone. Looking at actors that are not a part of the war had over a 150 journalists a part of casualties. Their deaths were to diminish the capacity to report the ongoing slaughter in the Balkan War (Collen 2021).

BALKAN ROUTE: WALKING TO SAFETY, A SOCIAL CHANGE

The Balkan Route is a past and present example of transgenerational trauma across diverse populations having women and children as the majority. The Bosnian women survivors of war crimes and war state their retraumatization with every story had on the same Balkan Route that they and their families traveled (KSW 2000–2022). The conclusion reached by the women is it is not that it will happen but is continual, an ongoing past present and future generations.

Again, the main challenge in data-sharing and metrics in identifying women and women refugees is that they do not have their life experiences that create culture and narratives in the technical improvements over decades; ethical, administrative, and bureaucratic policies and mandates outright firewalls significantly restrict the research (Katsanis 2023; Bibus and Carlsen 2015).

The requirement to have the both the place and space for psychosocial thriving skills, their life experiences, and the transgenerational trauma of their ancestors allows for cultural heritable information (Njaka and Peacock 2021; Villena-Mata 2022). Adaptive culture allows for the "place and space" intangible element: our physical environment directly influences emotions and well-being. The women survivors of war crimes and war who fled on the Balkan route and pathways with women refugees seek the flourishing, heritable skills to bond together and strive for a safe place for themselves and their families (KSW 2000–2022).

Seeking safety is an epigenetics tool of bonding since we heal "when the bond between a living thing and its world, the relationships we have with each other and our environment are the greater heredity force" (Anderson 2021; McTaggart 2011, 35). I found the best definition for epigenetics is an ancient Greek word meaning over and above our genome (National Human Genome Research Institute 2021). The epigenetic description indicates that women refugees' life experiences and narratives inform and allow them to author their lives toward safety—over and above their genome (Anderson 2021). Bonding in matrilineal culture and tacit knowledge are no longer invisible but are viable in times of crisis.

Bonding identified women refugees' tacit knowledge and that bonding with each other, and the environment is crucial for healing. Bonding interacts with the environment to influence our healing only when we know when to survive and thrive. The most primal urges—the bonding impulse—flow via the epigenetic transgenerational process when we act upon what matters and how we live and respond within our world (Lehrner and Yehuda 2018). Bonding impulses are a key epigenetic cultural psychological component of connecting and living (McTaggart 2011).

It was in the 1950s when psychologist John Bowlby devised attachment theory, which was originally focused on the infant-caregiver relationship (Ackerman 2018). Bowlby attachment theory cites that children come into the world biologically hardwired to form attachment bonds with others, but most of this work fails to center on the mother rather only in terms of caregiver and others. According to licensed clinical psychologist Angela Caron, "these attachment bonds are a primal survival mechanism" (qtd. in Volpe 2023).

Bonding is a movement meeting a host of influences within the family, the social collective, the status of relationships, and sense of fulfillment in life. In short, how one lives and and ones ancestors lived: the mother the most direct expression of our genome and thriving—the bonding for healing and how "epigenetics and adaptive evolution also display something remarkable about how we take physical form" (McTaggart 2011, 35). However, the South Slavic women survivors of war crimes and war and those who trudged on the Balkan Route and/or repatriation back to their homes if they were standing, the mothers, grandmothers recounted that none of the policies centered on them. According to the women survivors, they accepted that the target is their womb before, during, and after the wars and violence (KSW 2000–2022; Anderson 2015a). For them, it was a pivotal point to create an adaptive culture.

FEMALE BIOLOGY: MITOCHONDRIAL DNA-MTDNA—THE MISSING PIECE

Only recent genetic sciences revealed what is invisible in the male data sciences that her mitochondrial DNA-mtDNA is exclusively female—the mothers' egg is matrilineal in nature (Perez 2021). However, the sciences label mtDNA matrilineal as maternal inheritance instead of sourcing maternal inheritance as the origin of culture (Greiner et al. 2015). Ignoring the very complex female biological cultural totalities is a strategy of war and violence against women. What transcends upon maternal inheritance, cultural strengths to evolve, adaptability, human sociability health and overall flourishing inherent in healing transgenerational trauma is restricted to the maternal locality. The point where flourishing is critically needed to be self-sustaining and self-organizing (Wheeler 2006b, 40).

Another crucial point in the somatic biological and female biology as creators of evolving matrilineal culture is the mitochondria passed to children only by the mother (Cavalli-Sforza and Cavalli-Sforza 1993). Luigi Luca Cavalli-Sforza and Francesco Cavalli-Sforza (1993), authors of *The Great Human Diaspora*, dedicate their book to "women who gave us our mitochondria," since their research revealed that evolutionary female biology is about diversity and healing.

Cavalli-Sforza and Cavalli-Sforza (1993) write, "two children from the same mother will have identical mitochondria, even if the father is different. Every so often the mitochondrial DNA changes, or mutates, very slightly and one of the 16,500 nucleotides is replaced by another. From then on, all the descendants of that women will receive the mutated strand in its new form" (65). That rare phenomenon of mutation that occurs originates via epigenetic behaviors and life experiences adapting to the environment.

Culture begins with the somatic progression of biological felt states to mind/body experiences producing healing processes and reoccurring cultural interventions into future generations (Damasio 2018, 29). Damasio posits that "the crucial biological phenomena—feelings and intellect within cultural minds are only one part of the story. . . . At the same time, we need to recognize that the adaptations and faculties used by cultural minds were the result of natural selection and genetic transmission" (Damasio 2018, 29).

What is invisible or veiled to conceal matrilineal culture is referred to in Damasio's research and that of the male-biased sciences of the female biological phenomena is the heliocentric, how the sun is center for all planets orbiting (Perez 2021; Damasio 2018). What is meant here is the need and data required for sourcing of maternal inheritance as the center where life orbits. Thus, female biology- nature, the Slavic Moist Mother Earth for the women survivors of war crimes and war is the origin of culture and manifesting an adaptive culture (Hubbs 1993; Goueffic 2016).

Cavalli determined "Studying our origins and past helps us to understand ourselves. Much of our life depends on our cultural background—as well as on another fundamental factor, our genetic structure. Cultural transmission has not yet been analyzed in any depth. It is the factor that preserves cultural legacies through the generations and decides whether a custom or system is to stay or to go" (Cavalli-Sforza and Cavalli-Sforza 1993, 224).

But, with the rarity of female biology–inclusive research the question arises—what to do with a study by Mark Schoofs, a geneticist who determined "every person on Earth in our day can trace their lineage back to a common female ancestor and names her Mitochondrial Eve" (Asala 2020). The research of both Cavalli-Sforza and Cavalli-Sforza (1993) and Damasio (2018) on culture certainly places female biology as heliocentric, therefore women are the originators and creators of culture, a crucial medium from which to heal transgenerational trauma.

BLOCKING HOMEOSTASIS CATALYSTS

Since genetic tools regulate and synchronize life, a homeostasis, Damasio promotes "a working hypothesis on the relations between feelings and culture. Feelings as deputies of homeostasis are the catalysts for response that began human cultures" (Damasio 2018, 26). That working hypothesis for the South Slavic women survivors of war crimes and war understands feelings as being critical to flourishing right in the very minute of daily life. But the war survivors continue to endure femicide whenever addressing urgent crises, life-and-death situations (Anderson 2015a).

However, in the aftermath of the Balkan War, the women war survivors persist to move past fear moving from survival to thriving through their Slavic culture. When trauma is transgenerationally incited by violence, often by wars, survival does not move toward thriving or a human flourishing. But transformational change is where culture could provide the movement to flourishing (Green et al. 2003).

Since culture moves from survival to flourishing mechanisms, it gives rise toward creating the corresponding matrilineal oral memory traditions, a ritual memory science neurobiologically aligned to human sociality (Porges 2011; Wheeler 2006b). The informed trauma treatments with the women war survivors using their oral memory traditions and cultural practices house millennia-aged prevention tools, which are often discounted and overlooked by the sciences and the provision of humanitarian aid to governing entities (Ilieva and Shturbanova 1997; Perez 2021).

Wendy Wheeler (2006b), in her book *The Whole Creature: Complexity, Biosemiotics and the Evolution of Culture*, points to "an exclusive focus on reductionism and the mechanistic metaphor introduced by seventeenth-century European science . . . it is life and social sciences that have suffered most from this kind of approach" (29). As a result of science's reductionism and seventeenth-century mechanistic worldview, Slavic cultural life and social science matriarchal methods continue to be dismissed. Despite Slavic life and matriarchal feelings and behaviors that can pave an insight into the only possible prevention of infectious holocaustic femicide transgenerational trauma, it is excluded by the sciences and humanitarian agencies (Anderson 2015a; Perez 2021).

The informed trauma work with the women war survivors resulted in an important discovery, a problem statement; it is very apparent there continues to be very little data and narratives nor psychological or social sciences on the *impact* of women's trauma and how to resurrect healing of transgenerational trauma. The reality that the scientific categories of human lethal violence are a consensus of male data bias (patriarchal) despite the transgenerational role of men as predators is because data science "is overwhelming[ly] a male occupation" (Perez 2021, 2; Goueffic 2016).

You can find entire libraries of women's war crimes and war traumas in the role of victims or the deceased. Take for instance that Yugoslav International War Crimes Tribunal to prosecute war crimes as of 1995 did not have rape as a war crime (Copelon 1995). Two elements that are invisible is the impact this trauma has on women or how women are creators of culture that heals transgenerational trauma. The focus is on transgenerational trauma due to it being epigenetic—shaping and influencing our DNA through life experiences, a human sociality that is housed through culture (Wheeler 2006b; Damasio 2018).

Therefore, the rarity of studies and information on South Slavic women survivors of war crimes and war whose transgenerational trauma spans a century of wars—World War I, World War II, and the Balkan War—is not acknowledged and invisible in the sciences disregarded as a healing resource (Goueffic 2016; Mertus 2000). Instead, it is buried in sanctioned victim roles for women removing women's tacit knowledge (Green et al. 2003; Perez 2021; Goueffic 2016; Wheeler 2006b).

Only recently, the outcry for the inclusion of women in data sciences and the sciences has acknowledged the lethal violence women continue to endure. According to Caroline Criado Perez (2021), in her landmark book *Invisible Women: Data Bias in a World Designed for Men*, states, "the result of this deeply male-dominated culture is that the male experience, the male perspective, has come to be seen as universal, while the female experience—that of half the global population, after all—is seen as, well, niche" (12). The late Dr. Candace Pert (1999), an internationally recognized neuroscientist and pharmacologist who discovered the opiate receptor—the cellular binding site for endorphins—wrote that male-biased science is not open to another way of studying and understanding, therefore it is a trained incapacity, a patriarchal technological society.

The niche Caroline Criado Perez (2021) writes of is the invisibility of women in the data sciences and thus trauma that when studied belittle women's trauma and determined her female biology and trauma impacts to be insignificant. To have women feel insignificant results in women having no capacity to create a culture and homeostasis and indicates her fear and terror. According to the Bosnian women survivors, two factors that remarked how their lives did not matter (Anderson 2015b; KSW 2000–2022).

The first factor was that United Nations and humanitarian aid agencies and international military agencies carved borders since data on Bosnian women survivors of war crimes and war only existed in the terms of casualties or the victim status (Mertus 2000). The international aid and military allies governing entities funded the South Slavic males, whom the Bosnian women war crimes stated were only taking care of their own families and/or mafia criminals (Omerovic 2021).

Without their input or understanding of South Slavic culture, there was total erasure of women and internment in the victim role, which begat additional funding and military means that went to the same patriarchal infrastructure that exploded into the Balkan War, exploded into World War I, World War II, and the Ukraine War (2022) (Bahtijaragic and Pim 2015; Mertus 2000).

DAILY LIFE: THE EPIGENETICS OF TRANSGENERATIONAL TRAUMA HEALING

Cultural transmission in their Slavic Moist Mother Earth culture and oral memory rites encompasses all but deemed insignificant, worthless, or unpaid domestic labor (Mies 1998; Mertus 2000; Anderson 2015b). Worse yet, the Bosnian males would call the Bosnian women surivvors of war peasants or their bioculinary (life/culinary) herbs and food as medicine superstition or witchery (Anderson 2012a). Not having dinner on the table when the head of the household arrives home was reason enough to divorce her (KSW 2000–2022). To make matters worse, in Islamic religion, the Talaq Raji or Talq Bain (divorce), the husband only has to say I give you divorce (Religion of Peace 2023).

Despite the male's fear of her capacities to heal trauma to create a culture, homeostasis, and healing of trauma, the Bosnian women survivors of war as a women's collective at points defied the male-dominated dogma of violence and war. The women survivors of war became more conscious of having greater meaning and purpose when they participated in activism and regenerative practices such as growing self-sustaining gardens and marching for garage pickup in the aftermath of war (Anderson 2015a).

The finding in the research and two decades plus of clinical informed trauma is the Bosnian women war survivors' daily life—their personal life experiences and tacit knowledge in Slavic cultures is the spine of the consolidation of Slavic oral memory traditions (Anderson 2015a). The latter has epigenetic, thus transgenerational value toward healing transgenerational trauma.

Another significant piece of my research revealed that refugees are overwhelmingly women, mostly illiterate and poor globally, with few exceptions (Mertus 2000). Addressing women's trauma and issues prompts an urgent need to protect and restore sustaining the benefits that people derive from healthy adaptive and enabling cultural conditions including knowledge (Global Women's Institute 2017; Taub 2022). This is where the focus is needed in daily life since the minutia of life are targeted and disrupted by transgenerational violence from a century of wars.

Moving from feeling insignificance to significant through their daily life, the aftermath of a century of wars was intensified learning to overcome fear and terror through Slavic matriarchal cultural mandates (Schwartz 2018). The Bosnian women war survivors intuited that Slavic culture and the use of oral memory allowed the women to write their script— to be authors of healing transgenerational trauma and thus their lives (Anderson 2015b).

More importantly, the sciences are recognizing the value of daily life rituals intertwined with human sociability. Recently, in the bioarchaeological science investigating trauma and violence, a paper reports only a "often associated with social spheres of influence and power connected to daily life. Some forms of ritual violence also have restorative and regenerative aspects that strengthen community identity. Viewed in a biocultural context, evidence of osteological trauma provides rich insights into social relationships and the many ways that violence is embedded within those relationships" (Martin and Harrod 2015, 116). While the author does not give one indication that females are human or create biocultural context, she does acknowledge human sociability and the importance of oral memory traditions for daily life (Lienard and Boyer 2006; Damasio 2018).

Given the critical importance of healing women's trauma and women as the major caregivers and resource in wars and the aftermath of war it is perhaps surprising that women survivors are in a highly uneven global dataset (Murthy and Lakshminarayana 2006; Perez 2021). Since women are captured as indicators in the role of victims, not as a resource, researching for autopoietic, nonlinear approaches are unable, according to Wheeler, "to be phenomenologically embodied and embedded in culture and nature which must be seen as inextricably intertwined and codependent and coevolving" (Wheeler 2006b).

Access to gender-related factors is needed to maintain a strong focus on the local women who are the real experts and creators of culture. Women as a resource and not a target in violence and wars can assess the needs of the impacted population. Humanitarian efforts and the sciences should mainstream women at this point (Lafreniere et al. 2019; Mertus 2000).

Mentioned prior, during the two decades of informed trauma with Bosnian women survivors war, only one attempt to mainstream women as culture makers with the United Nations humanitarian effort for women was done. Surprisingly, but unknowingly, the United Nations incorporated the archaic ritual of dance in their Valentine's Day One Billion Rising project (Pollack 2013). What is important to note is that the UN response to a statistic that over a billion women will experience gender-based violence instigated the project (Pollack 2013).

Projects like One Billion Rising, which aim to address issues of violence and trauma, must ensure that women are not only recognized but actively involved in the healing process as agents of change and adaptive moving from resilience. By placing women at the center and valuing their experiences, skills, and contributions, these initiatives can foster a more comprehensive and inclusive approach to healing transgenerational trauma (Global Women's Institute 2017; Murthy and Lakshminarayana 2006).

By acknowledging and respecting women's agency and perspectives, patriarchal paradigms can be challenged and dismantled, creating a more balanced and supportive environment for healing and growth. When women are empowered as active participants in the healing process, they can emerge as strong leaders, nurturers, and advocates, contributing to the well-being of their communities and future generations.

It is crucial to recognize that healing from transgenerational trauma requires a collective effort that includes both women and men working together to create a more just and compassionate society. By embracing gender equality and promoting women's leadership, we can foster a more supportive and inclusive environment for healing and growth for all members of society.

Chapter 4

Maternal Fright

The chapter begins with a brief history of wartime effects on women. The lack of research on this population is made evident. The chapter's exploration of the history of wartime effects on women highlights the significant impact of conflict on this particular population. Psychosomatic approaches are discussed with a focus on the importance of taking gender-holistic approaches to treatment as well as accounting for cross-cultural differences.

In my search to heal trauma, I discovered that the Balkan War (1991–1994) dispersed and slaughtered many of my blood relations. Examining the impact of my family's transgenerational trauma, what arises is a homeostasis imperative, a code according to Antonio Damasio that is "aimed at the reduction of risks and dangers for individuals and social groups" (Damasio 2018, 29; Anderson 2015a). This led me to synthesize what many would call archaic knowledge of the structure of culture sociality and corresponding oral memory traditions—what is referred to as a ritual science (Anderson 2015a; Rubin 1995; Damasio 2018).

Cultural sociality incorporates the individual and collective intergenerational knowledge ritualized on the soma into a living body, somatic psychology, and a psycho-neurophysiological collective and communal cultural intergenerational knowledge (Lienard and Boyer 2006; Damasio 2018).

According to Pierre Lienard and Pascal Boyer (2006), ritualized behavior is based on the activation of a potential hazard as a precautionary response to present and future potential threats. Lienard and Boyer refer to ritualized behaviors activating the neurocognitive system and is highly effective to take the intuitive and to grasp the attention of the collective to pass on behavioral responses from one generation to another. As a result, the traumatic experiences, and the aftermath of trauma in the former Yugoslavia, may serve as a prototype for the planetary situation unfolding on a large scale. Take, for example, Russian aggression (2014 and 2022) in Ukraine that has resulted in war. Slavic cultured countries could set the stage for transgenerational wisdom replacing catastrophic transgenerational trauma and holocaustic transgenerational trauma (Steinmaurer et al. 2021).

For example, the Ukrainian war refugees in 2022, without a corporate, military, or humanitarian infrastructure somehow managed to have German, Polish, Moldavian, Romanian, Bulgarian—Balkan countries—women show up at rail stations to house them. One cannot pinpoint the media or any organization asking for these multinational women to do so. According to the South Slavic women war survivors, the response of women, mothers, and grandmothers was this incredible organic women's movement. It was a movement that these women learned from what happened in the Balkan, the Syrian, and the Afghan Wars, and from what happened to the African-to-Yemeni refugees on the Balkan Route (Kolo Sumejja Women [KSW] War Crimes and War Survivors 2000–2022).

Naming it as an emerging women's empowerment to carve out an adaptive culture triggered when daily life is disrupted and homes are either destroyed or in the middle of poverty surrounds or war zones, the women war survivors cite it is crucial to seeking safety in a relational place and space (KSW 2000–2022). Thomas Hubl (2020), author of *Healing Collective Trauma: A Process for Integrating Our Intergenerational and Cultural Wounds*, writes "those who choose to work directly with large groups in the service of collective trauma must be able to access cultural or ancestral material. This content is like a ghost in the room; it is invisible yet heavily felt" (48).

The South Slavic women war crimes and war survivors, and my mother, often said that when they had nothing, they found they had everything (Anderson 2015a). It speaks to an essence, an essential component of healing the trauma of the world, a world beset with chronic war and besieged by reckless governmental, humanitarian, and military leaders. Concentrated on women's transgenerational trauma, especially mothers and grandmothers, and all those who loved them when they "had nothing and had found everything," discovers the guiding human socially engaged healing process inclusive of tacit knowledge was to get on with the sustenance of life as best they could. That "everything" is what I define as culture, oral memory traditions, a South Slavic female human sociality healing transgenerational trauma.

When I first arrived at Sarajevo's old airport in 1999, it was still militarized with US-manned towers and tanks. As part of the nonprofit organization's (NGO's) education series for children, Medex Mine Awareness invited me to come and to heal the children's parents who were traumatized by the million-plus landmines in the region. At the airport, Medex's beat-up old car was painted with the NGO name on the car's rooftop. The reason for the signage on the roof was to identify it so as not be shot at or bombed from above. In the dilapidated NGO car with Bosnian music blaring and the driver singing, we followed right behind the US military convoy moving along the same route through the Bosnian mountains as they traveled to fulfill their mission to bomb Serbia.

In 1999, my first visit to the route from the old Sarajevo airport to Novi Travnik, a town that had experienced the ravages of war, provided a firsthand glimpse into the devastating effects of conflict on human lives and their cultural heritage. The scars of war are not only physical but also emotional, psychological, and deeply ingrained in the collective memory of communities that have endured such traumas. And this took place when simply *touring* the route from the old Sarajevo airport to the Croat and Muslim town Novi Travnik, just a half hour from the site of the 1984 Winter Olympics. Looking out the window of the car, I saw burned-out homes that were soaked and sagging beyond repair, demolished churches and mosques, decimated farms, hotels reduced to uninhabitable rubble, and roads that only a mountain goat could traverse. Nothing in the landscape was what Slavs have named as "Moist Mother Earth" (Hubbs 1993).

Upon arrival in Novi Travnik, however, a different sense came about. All the therapy tools from clinical psychology books, an office, a desk, scheduling consults, to trauma sessions were not plausible in conflict, whether it is due to domestic violence or to what occurs in war zones. It is in the collective, an emergence of human complexity, containing the reality of war crimes and war in the aftermath of wars, that leaves an unending physical and politically perilous war zone to this day (Steinmaurer et al. 2021). The aftermath of war is without human sociality—it's a constant survival.

Since few homes and buildings offered a space and place for therapies, let alone a safe place, socially engaged informed trauma therapies would mostly be conducted in open-air spaces where a million landmines were hidden, or in unsafe buildings that offered minimally a safe structure for orchestrating healing and warmth for the South Slavic women war survivors and me. The scarcity of food and wood for the stoves—*pech* in Serbo-Croatian—meant that in the brutal winters I would never take off my warm coats, gloves, and that I would sleep in my thermal underwear. I brought extra suitcases of food, seeds, and clothing, and left my own suitcase of clothes and toiletries in Bosnia. I would write my clinical notes with a battery-operated lamp at night near a woodstove and paid for the wood I used so I was not be a burden to the women survivors with whom I worked.

The donations given for the women of war crimes were largely spent on food and firewood for their families and the elderly living on the top floors of apartment buildings with destroyed elevators. Many elderly people died due to the extreme winters and the lack of food. Many times, I would ask of the few remaining humanitarian aid organizations or the Stabilization Force (SFOR) military what had happened to all the funding during the war and in the aftermath, since none of the women war survivors were receiving the much-needed help.

But somehow, I felt I had everything I would need; however, I could not put a definitive name to it. Of course, not having words is tacit knowledge and not to be dismissed—follow your hunches. Nor did my thumbing through psychology books and studies elucidate the fundamental element of Slavic female human sociality, an essentially social being prizing earth-based Slavic Moist Mother Earth interrelationships that move from survival to flourishing.

It was after that three-hour drive from the old Sarajevo airport that a paradigm shift began to occur. My attempts at making sense of the carnage allowed me to see more clearly the relationship between individual and culture and the use of South Slavic oral memory traditions used by the Slavic women war crimes and war survivors.

The South Slavic women, who had been survivors of war crimes and a century of wars, flourished by performing small acts carried out consistently and with great love. These women literally cleaned up before, during, and after the wars (Anderson 2015b; Bahtijaragic and Pim 2015). Traumatic events offer the soma, an intense multimodal learning, offering a thriving possibility that encourages ways of behaviors and which actions to perform. Babushka, elderly women with handmade brooms, swept up after the wars. Despite the invisibility, they baked sweets while boiling thick coffee in a wide-based and narrow-necked pot called a djesva—tasks carried out silently for generations, all behind the scenes of what was cited as momentous humanitarian aid and policies that did not support or recognize them (Mertus, Tesanovic et al. 1997).

As I observed old women staggering from carrying bags half their weight and mothers with infants and small children trudging past the men who sat hunched in cafanas drinking a thick demitasse of coffee, I realized that although this was in 1999, it could have been a scene from World War I or World War II (Anderson 2015a). The shattering transgenerational trauma—both emotional and physical—that I speak of and witnessed is read as the shattering experience that millions currently experience in many other global regions. This trauma also targets cultural healing processes where each new generation of children could have developed social cognition, cultural-epigenetic life experiences, and behaviors evolving in the face of the extant and wanton destruction of forests, rivers, species, and peoples—including children (Steinmaurer et al. 2021; Lafreniere et al. 2019).

Taking a closer look, the small acts and ritual of sweeping away the debris of war are the South Slavic oral memory traditions, behaviors, and responses adopted that move from survival behaviors to heal transgenerational trauma (Green et al. 2003). It is the South Slav's relationships with the "Moist

Mother Earth," encoded epigenetically, shaping, and influencing DNA (Anderson 2015b; Hubbs 1993).

These remnants of cultural practices, especially in women's everyday constant sustaining of life, are at the core of the healing process. The psychosomatic healing that exudes from the women's kolo rituals and oral memory tradition science of the Mesolithic folk round dancing and other practices are not easily captured by traditional empirical methods (Anderson 2015a). I describe it as the "women's evolutionary approaches surmounting what most would say are impassable obstacles and arduous struggles . . . ignored mainly by those humanitarian and justice agencies that were there to help" (Anderson 2015a; Green et al. 2003).

Despite worldwide media coverage of the Balkan War, the South Slavic women survivors of war crimes and war in the middle cantons of Bosnia and Herzegovina have received little attention. Yet, the women of a nation are undeniably the cornerstones for the continuation of life within and from that nation, not only in the reproductive sense, but also in terms of the intangible heritage that is shared with future generations (Martin and Harrow 2015; Jablonka and Lamb 2005). Jungian analyst Ester Harding (1997) noted that people, especially women in the modern era, have not honed their relationships with nature or evolved fear responses that enable survival in a world filled with global holocaustic trauma (Fromm 1973; Vlachovà and Biason 2004; D. S. Wilson 1994). In their book based on a United Nations report, Maria Vlachovà and Lea Biason (2004) explained, "We are confronted with the slaughter of Eve, a systematic gendercide of tragic proportions" (270). Clearly, the treatment of women in wartime has significant transgenerational repercussions for the survival of humanity (DeGruy 2017; Sarkissian and Sharkey 2021).

Maria B. Olujic (1998) argued that gendered violence is a gender-specific type of torture that is not only used in war, but also well-established in so-called peacetime. What exists in the literature, however, is an array of theoretical premises that ignore and exclude women's biological processes and omit the relationships and interconnectivity that arise from female social collectives, such as that of the South Slavic survivors (Allen 1996; Anderson 2015b; S. K. Fisher 1996; Christie and Pim 2012).

War crimes clearly affect females differently than males, both in terms of sexual victimization and in terms of survival rates as a result of physical trauma. However, it remains unknown how great the impact is on women's capacity to create culture and share collective memories in their roles as grandmothers, mothers, sisters, and daughters (Anderson 2015a; Steinmaurer et al. 2021).

FEMALE BIOLOGY: MATERNAL FRIGHT TRANSGENERATIONAL IMPACTS

For more than twenty years, working extensively with the Bosnian and Herzegovinian women war crimes and war survivors in the aftermath of the Balkan War (1991–1994), the South Slavic culture oral memory practices, the term maternal fright, *majka strah,* arose. When working with these survivors of war crimes, what became apparent was the incurred catastrophic wounding affecting perinatal and natal psychology and somatic impacts on both mother and child (Anderson 2015a; Porges 2007).

We need to understand the South Slavic women's disrupted sense of safety and realize the cost to their lives and to their children's lives (Anderson 2015a; Porges 2011). In fact, this is the very place where prevention and female solidarity flourish, eradicating maternal fright and securing safety for present and future generations (Anderson 2015a).

And who does not know of the Slavic Baba Yaga found in Russian and South Slavic intangible oral memory traditions? According to classical trained archaeologist Marija Gimbutas (1991), who cataloged thousands of zoomorphic bird goddess artifacts in the former Yugoslav region, the Slavic oral memory of Baba Yaga translated means "pelican" and "fright." Gimbutas's dynamic knowledge of archaeology combined with mythology, according to Joan Marler (1991), "provided a missing link for new understanding of European [and Slavic] prehistory" (1).

Many children's books of Vasilisa and Baba Yaga chronicle the use of oral memory of the orphaned girl child having in her apron pocket, a doll given to her by her deceased mother (Lang 2004). The girl child's apron pocket is symbolic of the womb (Hubbs 1993). Vasilisa's doll in her apron pocket would intuitively communicate to the direction she needed to take. According to Damasio (2018) "the constant sweep of our memories of past and future enable us in effect, to intuit possible meanings of current situations and to predict the possible future, immediate and not so immediate as life unfolds" (97). Vasilisa's intangible tacit knowledge can be in seen in how her mother line instructs the girl child to navigate the terrors of the dark forest to Baba Yaga's hut.

Given that the East Slavic story has Baba Yaga's hut erected and standing upon chicken legs and has a fence enclosure with skulls affixed at the top of the posts, Gimbutas understood that the zoomorphic artifacts and the folklore story of Vasilisa's doll and Baba Yaga's bird symbols were treasured and cultural transmissions as essential to life (Marler 1991). This oral memory story symbolizes the girl child's traumatic repercussions on the loss of her mother (Association for Psychological Science 2018).

My introduction to maternal fright was a thin Bosnian and Herzegovinian pregnant woman in her late twenties who had big dark circles under her eyes; her hands shook even at rest. When she began sharing her maternal fright, the words and her body poured iconic expressions into every physiological crevice that was once deliberately hidden and avoided. The fear and trauma are acute and chronic since the South Slavic, former Yugoslavian peoples have endured a century of wars, World War I, World War II, and Balkan War.

As previously discussed, my Serb mother was a World War II concentration camp survivor at Jasenovac (Anderson 2015a), and as a teen, she and her sister were assigned to the Ustashi Nazi SS Gradiska' pogrom. Both horrific and tragic, my mother's job was to toss the infants into the oven. As a result, when I had my two children, she refused to hold them as infants. The maternal fright was as apparent as it was during my childhood and into my adult years. She never talked about her experiences to me and most of this information was unknown to me until well after she died at the age of ninety. I have encountered similar patterns with South Slavic women in the aftermath of Balkan War, at a higher intensity (KSW 2000–2022).

I have determined maternal fright is the entrainment of transgenerational fear and trauma through female neurobiological processes (Anderson 2015a; Anderson 2014b; Christie and Pim 2012).

What I observed in the South Slavic women war survivors was that they focus on healing the impacts from violence. Strictly speaking, in the numerous interviews and sessions with the survivors, I noted how their healing impacts in response to violence do not follow the sequence listed and studied in historical and scientific pages for women war crimes and war survivors (Anderson 2015a).

Instead, with their looming maternal fright and the lack of medical and psychological response from helping aid organization to their maternal fright, prompted the war crimes and war survivors to produce a Slavic oral memory sequence of response to heal from violence which is focused on the consequences felt in the womb and corresponding interrelationships (S. K. Fisher 1996; Anderson 2015b; García-Muñoz et al. 2014).

What was observed is a social engagement system, human sociability, described in Stephen Porges's (2007) polyvagal theory, which is held in the South Slavic oral memory traditions and culture—where culture is created by women due to their biological process of menses, pregnancy, birth, and childrearing (see also Damasio 2018). Given that culture and oral memory traditions are epigenetic in nature, recent studies support that the Bosnian women war survivor's assessment of transgenerational impacts are from stress and from fear/fright (Babenko et al. 2015).

According to scientist Olena Babenko (2015), her clinical study revealed,

> recent human epidemiological and animal studies indicate that stressful experiences in utero or during early life may increase the risk of neurological and psychiatric disorders, arguably via altered epigenetic regulation. [It is] prone to changes in response to stressful experiences and hostile environmental factors. Altered epigenetic regulation may potentially influence fetal endocrine programming and brain development across several generations. Only recently, however, more attention has been paid to possible transgenerational effects of stress. We propose that prenatal stress, through the generation of epigenetic alterations, becomes one of the most powerful influences on mental health in later life. The consideration of ancestral and prenatal stress effects on lifetime health trajectories is critical for improving strategies that support healthy development and successful aging. (Babenko et al. 2015)

Their focus is on corresponding interrelationships whereby fundamental biological processes are joined with neurobiology, physiology and somatic psychology, and somatic movement therapies and concerns gestation-pregnancy. The reasoning proffered by both the women survivors of war crimes and war was universally stated as the key for generating healing functionality. But, more specifically, the survivors added a very finely detailed feature, the key to the interrelationships is the inclusiveness of female biology and nature and as women creators of culture and oral memory traditions (Porges 2011; Wheeler 2006b; Anderson 2015a; Silva 2014; Porges 2001).

The reason stated by the survivors being so attuned to female biology and to cultural nurturance was the proliferation of fear and trauma that has taken over their oral memory traditions and their capacity to manifest culture. Seen from the standpoint of what they had lived—their life experiences for the past three generations—their female biological processes such as menstruation and pregnancy to birth are targets for violence (forced pregnancies, rapes) and wars. The war survivors remarked constantly about life's agency explaining how living systems need to behave as nature and biology do in order to heal in the deeper sense (Anderson 2015a; Hoffmeyer 2008).

Biosemiotican Wendy Wheeler describes the functional structure of tacit knowing as "internalizing knowledge of the parts so that we can 'get' the whole" (Wheeler 2006b, 63). Wheeler states semiotician Polyani includes phenomenal structure in tacit knowing as the knowledge of the whole allows us to know more about it.

More importantly, what I encountered in these women was their female tacit knowledge that the roots of culture are biological and neurologically aligned with movements found in the life experiences of ancestors and the mother's life (Wheeler 2006b). In this regard, we are able to ascertain how mothers' embodied manifestation and transmission of culture, such as the perinatal states and child rearing, are based upon female corporeality that cannot be separated from their life experiences, thus shaping our DNA and gene state expressions (Sarkissian and Sharkey 2021; Jablonka and Lamb 2005; Rossi 2002; Merleau-Ponty 1995/1968).

I need to define the term maternal fright from a female tacit knowledge approach (Hoffmeyer 1996; Polanyi 1966). Female tacit knowledge represents "the bodily roots of our knowledge to [wom-] man highest creative powers" (Polanyi 1966, 15) based on the biological fact that we all are born of a woman, Maternal fright is an outcome of escalating man-made conflicts, wars, and violence. The female body and womb are targets of bodily assaults ranging from harm and sexual assaults/rapes to femicide, the mass murder of females. The victimized woman's stories and life experiences of violence perpetrated as a victim are the only expression allowed and studied.

However, her female tacit knowledge is disavowed as nonsensical, if not superstitions, and not grounded in fact and reality. Certainly, female tacit knowledge is not included in biological, medical, or scientific studies since the divisive difference is best acknowledged by scientist Helen E. Longino (2002) who wrote "men occupy a position of entitlement to women's bodies" (Pérezes 2021; Longino 2002).

Given that maternal fright erupted from the ongoing violence, the way violence has succeeded to be transgenerational is through the South Slavic female cultural transmission oriented perinatal oral memory practices (Damasio 2018; Anderson 2014b; 2015b; Christie and Pim 2012). Because oral memory traditions and practices are based on our ancestors' lived daily lives preserved and moved forward into future generations, the repeating behaviors shape genetic expression over generations (Steinmaurer et al. 2012; Kida 2014; University of California 2022). What is at hand here within oral memory traditions is the applied translation of our body's biological and neural code (Wheeler 2006b; Porges 2007; Hoffmeyer, 2008).

There are three properties of oral memory traditions. The first property is to manifest culture that is shown through the perinatal states, the development of the fetus and child-rearing, and future generations. Basically, the perinatal stages are the emergence of life with the encircling biological self-organizing membranes (Wheeler 2006b). Researcher Sue Gerhardt (2006) study pointed to babies as a genetic blueprint where the baby and the nurturing care given is an inseparable whole.

The second is to evolve through repeating practices honed on behaviors and movement that shape our DNA. What we are talking about concerns heritable generational significance and a retrocausality where influences from the present generation allow for change along with transgenerational epigenetic influences in neurogenetics that connect multiplex pedigrees of how behavior and stimuli respond to external stimuli (University of California 2022; Hubl 2020). And three, oral memory traditions proliferate in what Chris Knight's

(2013) *Blood Relations: Menstruation and the Origins of Culture* names as culturgens or memes mapping of cultural units (see also Levinson 2006).

You can say oral memory traditions are centered on female collective evolution since female biological process coupled with the discovery of memories are passed down through behavioral changes adjusting genetic expression to change our DNA. South Slavic oral memory traditions and practices have transgenerational knowledges' propensity to evolve by layering each generation's repeating behaviors to move from surviving to thriving (Barr and Skrbis 2008).

It is the transgenerational nature of perinatal oral memory practice, and its corresponding gestational vulnerability, that have become the targets of wars and violence. Thus, the South Slavic women survivors, as a female collective, are grappling with the psychobiological and neurobiological impacts of trauma in order to transform the transgenerational gynocidal implications with their oral memory practices (Anderson, 2014b; 2015b; Christie and Pim, 2012).

This absence of healing practices due to trauma impacts is noted in the somatic psychology field, Pat Ogden and Kekuni Minton (2000) study titled "Sensorimotor Psychotherapy: One Method for Processing Traumatic Memory" have found the "the traditional psychotherapy addresses the cognitive and emotional elements of trauma but lacks the technique that work directly with physiological elements, despite the fact that trauma affects the body and many symptoms of traumatized individuals are somatically based" (149).

According to Yi-Fu Tan, the gestating female is "if space allows movement, place is a pause and body is 'lived body' and space is humanly construed space" (quoted in Christie and Pim 2012, 287). How the young and pregnant woman war survivor knew that Mother Nature is hard at work to take and form habits describing the agency involved in biosemiotics, especially in the epigenetic and neurobiology science, is phenomenal. Given, her understanding and female tacit knowledge that the womb is a female humanly construed space, the South Slavic women's biosemiotics, epigenetic and neurobiology foci show the body instructing the mind (Christie and Pim 2012, 285).

Since Biosemiotics, epigenetics and neurobiology, and life/signs of life/life of signs have a perinatal universal validity, we can relate to the term of semiosphere coined by semiotician Yuri Lotman, a Russian-born Estonian (see Hoffmeyer 2008). Jesper Hoffmeyer (2008) quotes Brooke Williams from the Semiotic Society of America, who states every movement needs a symbol to grow. "A sign of a sign, the caduceus, the staff of a messenger bearing a message."

The biosemiotican Jesper Hoffmeyer (2008) termed biosemiotics as the name of an interdisciplinary scientific project that is based on the recognition that life is fundamentally grounded in semiotic processes (3). The semiosphere is a known cultural concept since the semiosphere is the semiotic unit of measure with the outcome in the development of culture—the totality and organic whole of living matter and the conditions for the continuation of life (Verdansky 2012). The semiotic unit of measure is mirrored in the applied oral memory traditions and practices (Lotman 2000). For example, author Mary Elizabeth Husslein (2013) in her research studied patterns in the oral memory traditions, the Gregorian chant melodies, where the meter self-organized into mensural units giving the chants a pulse.

Oral memory traditions are fundamental for South Slavic memory practices because the somatic psychobiology and biosemiotics (inclusive gestalt) involve "actions created, repeated, reproduced and elementally charged through meaningful agency" (Christie and Pim 2012, 287).

MATERNAL FRIGHT HEALING PRACTICES RESPONSES

The young pregnant woman war survivor, rubbing her swollen belly, understands her womb is the space and place of targeted violence, thus producing what South Slavic women name as maternal fright. And she has good reason; maternal fright is transgenerational and uniquely sensitive to fear and to the resulting traumas. Before the epoch of man-made violence, natural disasters and life's crises were the only intensified learning environments as transgenerational epigenetic purveyors of South Slavic oral memory traditions that manifested a culture of thriving and not just a surviving mechanism. However, with violence, culture and the applied oral memory traditions for thriving are consumed and face destruction as a result of the modern era of fear, fright, and trauma.

Maternal fright is contagious, the Bosnian and Herzegovinian pregnant woman tells me, pointing to my shaking hands (Anderson 201b5; Christie and Pim 2012). I had just finished an intense learning session with the communities' elder women, which involved dancing kolo and feasting. The women directed me to go to the pregnant woman's apartment immediately afterward.

Staring out of the window, she shares with me how her husband lost eighteen relatives in the Ahmica-Vitez genocide on April 16, 1993 (Anderson 2015b, Christie and Pim 2012). Her husband's family lived in a farming community and "on April 16, 1993, 150 Muslims in Ahmica-Vitez, mostly elderly and children as young as infants, were slaughtered by Croatian military war criminals during the Muslim early call to prayer" (Anderson 2014b, Christie and Pim 2012). While the young couple lives in Novi Travnik, Bosnia, around five kilometers away, it appears that the inflicted trauma effortlessly roams across vast distances and into future generations.

After an hour of sharing how she felt that her husband's fears were affecting her pregnant womb-environment—thus the fetus—the expecting mother asked what to do to protect her unborn child from her maternal fright. Her next movement is second nature for Slavs in that she was seeking a tradition or ritual to practice. Since, there was no oral memory practice to prevent an unborn child from the transgenerational trauma of maternal fright that resulted from violent genocide, gynocide, and rapes during the war, she was about to create a ritual to fill the void.

When she took a green magic marker that I had placed on the kitchen table with an art pad in the beginning of her sharing, I thought she was going to draw what she could not say in words—her tacit knowledge. But instead of drawing on the art paper, she used the green marker to draw a spiral on her pregnant belly. Starting from her belly button, she carefully and slowly etched the spiral in concentric circles, enveloping her swollen belly. When she finished, she pronounced what appears to be Slavic thaumaturgy—embodied miracle making—that she had added a new ritual and practice to the Slavic oral memory traditions to eradicate maternal fright.

Of course, the pregnant woman war survivor did not know of the classically trained Lithuanian archaeologist Marija Gimbutas, who describes the former region of Yugoslavia to be the evolution and symbolic communication that it was the cradle of the spiral art (Gimbutas 1991, 56; Marler 1991). Harald Haarmann (1997), a linguist, reports that the script, such as the Old Europe spiral, are evolutive continuity and "is a typical feature in setting where original cultural patterns evolve continuously and form a trend without disrupter or major disturbances" (108).

I have observed many Bosnian mothers and their children unable to circumvent the transgenerational trauma or to eradicate maternal fright. More than twenty years after the Balkan War in Bosnia and Herzegovina, many young children display transgenerational trauma as if they had been alive during the war. Through the years, I was involved with projective art for grammar school. The children's pictures often showed guns, murdered family members, and dismembered bodies, and I wondered how these young children could know of the violence that was in past.

What I am witnessing is epigenetic transgenerational maternal fright; children relive their mothers' traumatic life experiences. According to Joy DeGruy (2017), clinical psychologist, and author of the book *Post Traumatic Slave Syndrome: American's Legacy of Enduring Injury and Healing*, she noted that there was the inherent, if not learned, Black Slavery post-traumatic stress syndrome, "an anthropological assertion and lived experiences of our ancestors" (quoted in Clemmons 2020).

Considering that mothers pass down both epigenetic influences as well as oral traditions onto their children, it is not surprising that, in the world of violence, that maternal fright, which affects gene expression and is set in memory, is passed down the generations (Kaitz et al. 2009). The reality of violence against women, a conveyor of maternal fright, is embedded in the infrastructure of wars, domestic violence, sexual assault, and homicide (Sarkissian and Sharkey 2021; Global Women's Institute 2017; Wood 2006; Krug et al. 2002).

All have catastrophic statistics but one US statistic that stands out is that the leading cause of death for pregnant mothers is trauma that involves strangulation, most often committed by their partners (Falb et al. 2014; Fildes et al. 1992). According to the 2011 statistic reporting, the seventh leading cause of death for women is femicide; mass murder of women (J. S. Wilson et al. 2011; van Wormer and Roberts 2009). For African American women and Native American women, femicide is the second leading cause of death (J. S. Wilson et al. 2011). When you look at wars, the escalating civilian fatalities since World War II are mostly women and children, and the battlefield is in wombs and homes (Mertus and Benjamin 2000). These statistics suggest that maternal fright is a common occurrence across diverse ethnic groups (Amoakohene 2004).

However, due to the inherent male bias (Perez 2021) in statistics, according to the femicide report, "collecting correct data on femicide is challenging, largely because in most countries, police and medical data-collection systems that document cases of homicide often do not have the necessary information or do not report the victim–perpetrator relationship or the motives for the homicide, let alone gender-related motivations for murder. However, data on the nature and prevalence of femicide are increasing worldwide" (World Health Organization (WHO) 2012).

I observed the epigenetics of trauma in one young Bosnian child, around five years of age, who was standing in the small playground at the bottom of a dull, war-weary apartment building. She stood alone in the playground as if frozen, with a posture assumed by many parents who stand alone and watch the children play. Her father noticed me looking at his daughter, walked over to me, and started sharing what happened to the child's mother. One early morning, soon after he left for work, his wife jumped from their flat's tiny balcony to the pavement below. Her daughter was a few months old when her mother flew off the balcony. None of the neighbors knew what had happened, which meant that the infant was alone for hours before the mother's body was noticed on the apartment building's woodpile. Immediately after being notified, the father went to check on his infant. The daughter was so exhausted from crying and hunger. He said that she was very desperately quiet and not moving, frozen from the cold apartment.

The father went on to state that his wife's death was listed as an accident. But he said he has heard of too many accidents of tripping off the flat's balconies to believe that it was. He asked why a young mother would leave her daughter and him. Many mothers in Novi Travnik and Travnik, the four-thousand-year-old Bird Goddess artifacts strewn in the former Yugoslavia, flew off their balconies to their deaths. All were listed as accidents according to the father.

As if to corroborate the father's statement, every one of my interviews over the past twenty years with the families whose mother, wife, female caregiver died from "accidental tripping off balconies and windows" reported the same disbelief of naming their deaths as accidental (Anderson 2015a).

What I noted in more than two decades of fieldwork is that in Bosnia and Herzegovina, the women survivors of war crimes and war, in response to the "accidental deaths" of mothers leaping to their deaths, enacted an orchestrated movement to have the balconies filled with flowers and vegetables no matter how small. When I interviewed the women survivors about what I was observing, I was told about the oral memory traditions of bringing food at the funeral and memorials as it was a South Slavic and, also, an Islamic practice.

The flowers draping and flowing over the pockmarked bullet and grenade holes on or near the balconies would have vines and flowers covering the balconies and apartment's wounds. The elder of the Kolo (circle) Sumejja women survivors from Novi Travnik, Bosnia and Herzegovina, cited, "never underestimate the flowers and plants to prevent the leaps, there's no space for their feet and we do not step on plants" (Anderson 2012a).

ORAL MEMORY TRADITIONS ARE EPIGENETIC

With oral memory traditions, we are talking about the epigenetic behaviors producing social engagements, once repeated, and lived daily, continue to be practiced in future generations (Cowan et al. 2021). A new field, behavioral epigenetics, is catching up to the tacit knowledge—we know more than we can tell—in oral memory traditions. The emphasis is on memory, thus on epigenetics (Kandel 2007).

In following research in epigenetics and in memory, a recent study indicates that the transmission of epigenetic memory occurs across multiple generations (University of California 2022). Susan Strome, professor emerita of molecular, cellular, and developmental biology at the University of California Santa Cruz (2022) states "the once radical idea that such changes in gene expression can be inherited now has a growing body of evidence behind it, but the mechanisms involved remain poorly understood." The use of oral memory traditions by the South Slavic women survivors of war crimes and war would not be called radical, and through tacit knowing the Bosnian War survivors understand the epigenetics and the memory behind it.

In considering biosemiotics, bio-life, and semiotic signs, we can further connect all of the vast interrelationships of nature/nurture with biology (Wheeler 2006b). Moshe Szyf, a molecular biologist, and Michael Meaney, a neurobiologist, in their study of nature or nurture, biology or psychology concerning why behaviors are developed and persist through the generations, considered a hypothesis: "If diet and chemicals can cause epigenetic changes, could certain experiences—child neglect, drug abuse, or other severe stresses—also set off epigenetic changes to the DNA inside the neurons of a person's brain?" (qtd. in Hurley 2013, 51).

But, more importantly, the South Slavic oral memory traditions have known somatic (living body) psychology and psychobiology reveal a psychobiological pathway that appears to point to some of the mechanisms underlying the interplay of a gene-environment transactional approach related to neurobiological processes (Porges 2011; Bentz et al. 2013; McGowan et al. 2008).

Our ancestors' experiences found in oral memory traditions have never seen the scale of increasing volume of violence against female bodies and gestation. Given how you and I live life today, and that today's life will be lived by our grandchildren, this theory presents essentially a way to heal trauma and eradicate violence. The South Slavic women survivors are facing a crisis in that as creators of culture and having the oral memory practices devoid of ways and means to rid maternal fright sets up seemingly impossible obstacles. However, the epigenetic transgenerational nature of oral memory traditions has provided the survivors a platform to discover meaning in catastrophic trauma and practices that halt violence (Anderson 2015b; Damasio 2018).

MATERNAL FRIGHT IS COMMON IN MODERN WARS AND VIOLENCE

The Slavic term "maternal fright" is carved into our modern era of man-made wars and violence, and is a common consequence of the forgotten conflict, the Balkan War (1991–1994) in the former Yugoslav region (Anderson 2015b; Christie and Pim 2012; deMause 2006). Maternal fright can be traced to prehistoric times (Baring and Cashford 1991; Gimbutas 1991). Traumatic events and natural disasters or crises that occurred in prehistoric eras resulted in survival memories, which ensured the species' survival across generations. In modern times, survival memories are a result of a world of violence and wars (Buss and Plomin 2014). It has been proposed that epigenetic processes have shaped human DNA from prehistoric times to the present and that maternal survival memories are heritable in this way (Jablonka and Raz 2009).

Maternal fright inflicts transgenerational anxiety disorders and a host of mental and physical illnesses, which especially impact the perinatal and early life development of the child. But, what needs to be considered with femicide is the cost involved when maternal nurturing and transgenerational memories are eradicated due to violence (Babenko et al. 2015; Singer et al. 2003). For the South Slavic women in particular, the century of wars and war crimes (World War I, World War II, and Balkan War) has led to maternal fright becoming a part of their oral memory traditions and practices, possibly to ameliorate the devastating impacts of trauma.

CHILDREN REMEMBER WHAT THEIR MOTHER REMEMBERS

Mother's experiences have a profound effect on the development and the life of a child (Hesse and Main 1999; Wadhwa 2005). These experiences are passed on to the child through oral traditions that relay events and experiences through social interactions (Kaitz et al. 2009; Schore 2001). In addition, epigenetic processes, which are influenced by maternal experiences and environment, therefore, affect gene expression of the fetus (Bentz et al. 2013; University of California 2022; Champagne 2010).

Given that the transmission of maternal life experiences and memories shapes our species' genes and behavior, we can observe how maternal daily life experiences and those repeated over time are preserved in oral memory traditions, and how a science of rituals plays into biological rhythms and cycles. All the tacit knowledge and life experiences are passed down to future generations orally, daily life-epigenetics, and through influencing and shaping our genes (Greiner et al. 2015; Wheeler 2006b, Polanyi 1962). For instance, we know that babies have a programmed inherited fear and instincts (Hodgson 2004).

Slavic oral memory traditions are centered on the mother of the Slavic Moist Mother Earth (Anderson 2015b; Christie and Pim 2012; Slapšak 2005). Mothers aid in the transmission of culture by knowing when to survive and when to employ thriving skills through chants, dance, bioculinary practices, and art (Anderson 2015b; Steinmaurer et al. 2021; J. L. Hanna 1987; Parncutt 2009). By communicating with the infant, the mother maternal influences the child's language capacity and the resulting mega-library of ancestors' life experiences and memories (University of California 2022; Bates 2014).

Estela V. Welldon (1992) purported that the quality of female biology and body is critical for women's psychology, explaining how violence and wars target female biology and bodies, since women birth their own creations (see also Fonagy 2010). For much of one hundred years of World War I, World War II and the Balkan War in the former Yugoslav region, the women survivors led their domestic lives and performed repetitive acts that sustained them and their families (Anderson 2015b; Christie and Pim 2012).

As a result, their South Slavic oral memory traditions from a psychobiological perspective proliferated a variety of practices and traditions that aimed to heal and to prevent maternal fright from infecting future generations (Anderson 2015a).

Oral memory traditions, such dance, songs are preserved and perpetuated encouraging social engagements into the community and future generations to evolve and adapt to their environment (Green et al. 2003; S. K. Fisher 1996; Levy and Sznaider 2006; Steiner and Zelizer 1995). The practices are rooted in biology. According to Damasio (2018, 95–96), "singing a song with lyrics requires the time-locked integration of varied fragments of recall: the melody that guides the singing, the memory of the word, the memories related to motor execution (Damasio 2018, 95–96). The Slavic oral memory traditions include chants, dance, and agricultural, culinary, herbal, and medicinal practices.

During the Balkan War and in the aftermath, this knowledge of the environment, nature, and the land saved many from death and diseases. Take the folk round dance, called the kolo, meaning wheel or to be in a circle, social engagement (Anderson 2015b; Ilieva and Shturbanova 1997; Allen and Hubbs 1980; Hubbs 1993). Ilieva and Shturbanova cite that "one of the main functions of the ritual dance in folklore cultures is to covey knowledge: knowledge about the structure of the world, about how to live in community, self-knowledge, knowledge about the order, laws and government of society and knowledge of a mythological world view" (Ilieva and Shturbanova 1997, 309–10). The kolo is Mesolithic in age, and the Laban-Bartenieff system dance movement and movement psychotherapy have mapped the kolo patterns and rhythms in tandem with the affective neuroscience work of Steven Porges and polyvagal regulation (Eddy 2009; Homann 2010; Porges 2011). Porges, mapping the nervous system, identifies the vagus, the tenth vagus cranial nerve, as contributing to self-regulation, an internal viscera that includes the heart but relates to autonomic function to behaviors and movement (Porges 2011).

This led my clinical trauma research on female biology to include menstruation cycles and to consider how the kolo oral memory rites folk round dances, or to be in a circle for Slavs, birthed social engagements as a collective (Anderson 2015a). The finding that there were no significant menstrual changes from during to after the war suggests that the oral tradition practice of the kolo has healing properties, providing the women with an intermediate space from which the female body interacts with the locus of culture. Thus, on the basis of menstruation, maternal care, childbirth, and survivorship of war crimes and war experiences, the intermediate functioning of the potential space occurs via the body, corporeality, language, images, and shared symbols.

The sample of war crimes and war women survivors had had continuous exposure to each other in the aftermath, rather than during the war, in which many were refugees were fleeing from violence. Some aspect of the kolo indicates a healing ritual via the embodiment of female roles during traumatic events. The oral memory traditions, as a practice, do not ensue via cognition but through a multisensory or synesthetic bodily experience, through the sharing of the women's war crimes and war experiences (Anderson 2015a; Porges 2007). More importantly, the sensorium in both physical and mental illness is organized, despite female war victims being at the edge of public order and often invisible to helping aid agencies.

Therefore, oral memory traditions are a supporting infrastructure that house embedded somatic psychological and physical movements to incorporate the whole body/mind/culture. This may be one possible reason that the women may not have experienced menstrual changes from during and after the war due to their use of the oral memory traditions of the kolo. Field notes support the premise of the kolo activity as their only supporting infrastructure, since the war crimes and war survivors reported their invisibility in the eyes of aid organizations and the Stabilization Force (SFOR) policies.

"We had nothing. I shared a spoon with eight of us for what food we had. The kolo organized us seamlessly," reported the female leader of the kolo, a member of the women war survivors' group. Additionally, the survivors reported that their menstrual periods became more synchronized and closer together with their kolo and circle activities. But more importantly, the healing of trauma took place within the social formation of the kolo oral memory traditions (Anderson 2014a; Ilieva and Shturbanova 1997).

Since the female war crimes and war survivors were invisible and neglected by the helping aid agencies, their only supportive infrastructure was their Mesolithic kolo that filled in the gap (Anderson 2014a; Ilieva and Shturbanova 1997). The Mesolithic kolo is an inherently female humanities and culture manifestation that occurs during pregnancies, birth, and the raising of children. War and its atrocities targeted female civilians and their children and continues to do so in the aftermath of wars. Thus, the kolo, indigenous to the survivors of war crimes and war, offered much-needed support and healing for the women's acute and chronic trauma situations during the war and in the aftermath (Christie and Pim 2012; Mertus 2000).

Given the consistent kolo and circle activity during the Balkan War and in the aftermath, the regularity of menstrual cycles is explained. Memory danced, or in the circle, according to the South Slavic women war crimes and war survivors, is a socially engaged collective intelligence (Anderson 2012a; Christie and Pim 2012; Hershey et al. 2014). In terms of the goal of this thesis to search for trauma interventions, kolo's social intelligence allots representations of space and spatial data from which to archive cultural social memory in order to provide a biological ecology and human sociability proffering a sense of safety (Wheeler 2006b; Hershey et al. 2014).

It stands to reason with the oral memory traditions practices focused on an inheritance system, with genetic, epigenetic, behavioral, and the symbolic, to carve intergenerational memories that Kandel's (2006) research, which defines trauma as memory disorders, would be interfacing each other (Jablonka and Lamb 2005, 235). The Mesolithic kolo, as an applied somatic psychology practice, heals traumatic memory in a social collective by archiving the memories and layering over the memories to heal or to pass down thriving skills and adaptive skills. More importantly, healing trauma also heals biological impacts, such as menstruation, for female war crimes and war survivors.

For example, the South Slavic kolovodja folk dance is contingent on a female social collective movement relating to the autonomic nervous system—its affective experience—linking emotional expression and vocal communications in the chants and songs sung while dancing the kolo (UNESCO 2017; Anderson 2014a; 2015a; Porges 2007; Christie and Pim 2012). The vodja, known as the female guide who narrates (communicates) chanting the continuous archives of the dance through bodily cues, is done to introduce step changes and rhythms igniting new patterns in kolovodja folk dance, thereby transforming fear and terror into feeling safe (Porges 2007; Ronström 1991).

SOCIAL COLLECTIVE CAN HEAL MATERNAL FRIGHT

The African saying, "it takes a village to raise a child," expresses the female social collective and interrelated female kinships that serve as evidence that the cultural environment influences development (Asala 2020; Rosaldo and Lamphere 1974; van Anders 2014). The female social collective includes men, never excludes women, and remembers the children (I. M. Young 1994). Imprisoned women, whether in penal systems, rape war camps, refugee camps, or patriarchal infrastructure held in isolation, often lack this social collective of transgenerational traumas healing due to their entrenched survival mechanisms (Green et al. 2003). Traumatic events associated with these imprisonment conditions are transgenerational survival mechanisms as opposed to flourishing epigenetic processes.

For the South Slavic Bosnian women survivors of war, memories have been carved from violent epochs and perhaps, a healing element will be passed to future generations. Of the three million refugees from the Balkan War who left with nothing but a suitcase, 80 percent were women (Mertus et al. 1997). This high concentration of women resulted in a vast Slavic female social collective that can institute beginning steps to heal maternal fright (Anderson 2015a; Mertus 2000).

For example, in 2022, the Ukraine War had the estimate of the percentage of refugees refugees ranging from 90 percent to 98 percent of the refugees (Taub 2022). In the Balkan War, some three million refugees were estimated to flood Europe, with 75 percent to 80 percent being women (Mertus 2000). Both represent a vast female social collective. The Slavic female social collective, in the case of the Ukrainian women fleeing to Poland, had Polish women form an organization Kobiety za Kolko—Women Take the Wheel (Kakissis 2022). Noting the interconnection of Balkan and Slav languages, this overlaps with the word origin and meaning for the Slavic folk round dance or circle—wheel is found in the Polish word Kolko.

It is not surprising with the Slavs that the Polish "Women Take the Wheel" organization had women drivers who would make regular trips to the war zone. The war zoner border is also a sex-trafficking-infested border. Since the meaning of the word "kolo" to mean the wheel—movement, circle—the Polish women's humanitarian movement effort took the women war victims to be either reunited with their families or taken to homes and shelters. The United Nations had a table at the rail station with information but could not give any resources to the fleeing Ukrainian women. However, the female social collective in Poland and in Germany stepped in (Blair 2022).

Members of the Polish and German female social collective were arriving daily at the rail stations and housing the Ukrainian women refugees. In fact, maternal human sociability was evident at the Przemusl train station, where the Polish female collective left strollers, bags filled with essentials, and stuffed animals for the fleeing Ukrainian women and children (Blair 2022).

Julie Mertus, in 1997, was taken aback with the Bosnian women war crimes and war survivors, with their invisible and untouched narratives unless the women were victims—it prompted her book titled *The Suitcase: Refugee Voices from Bosnia and Croatia* (Mertus et al. 1997).

The Bosnian women war survivors with regard to the Ukrainian War refugees (2022) see themselves in the fleeing Ukrainian women refugees. In fact, the Bosnian War survivors voiced their retraumatization (KSW 2000–2022). Some of the participants, the older ones, said they did their work and now it is time for the younger ones to step in. The Bosnian War survivors said it was not that they were too busy raising grandchildren, but also the fact that their adult children are flung across the world after the Balkan War in the diaspora (KSW 2000–2022). The most common response was that it is not safe in Bosnia and Hercegovina due to the political situation that will cause another war in former Yugoslavia.

MATERNAL FRIGHT CAN CHANGE A CHILD'S GENES

In the modern age, trauma induced by conflicts, wars, and armed violence affects the epigenetic processes, thus targeting women's capacity to manifest culture. Culture's roots are biological, as is the mother. Her uterine endowments are absent from the male body, and her uterus as an organ is wholly female. The uterine endowments are such as to carry intricate biological processes interconnected with emotional states and cues to fight-or-flight responses. What is understood about the uterine environment is that the fight-or-flight response ensures the survival of the species but, more importantly, that the transmission of maternal life experiences and memories shapes gene expression in future generations toward evolving thriving with adaptability (Kaitz et al. 2009; Hesse and Main 1999; Hastie 2008).

Maternal fright resulting from man-made violence leads to epigenetic inheritance of negative experiences. The environment of war and violence can influence genetic variability factors passed from the mother to the child, leaving a legacy of mental and health impacts (Van den Bergh et al. 2005). Just as the uterine environment is fragile and absorbingly pliable, the world the mother resides in also influences the interplays of plasticity found in biology, nurture, and nature.

A child's development and gene expression are sensitive not only to the uterine environment, but also to the maternal environment and her life experiences. Maternal fear and anxiety pose a risk of serious physical and mental problems for both the mother and the child (Van den Bergh et al. 2005). It has been shown that the mother's anxiety and stress that elicit strong emotional experiences can increase the risk for spontaneous abortion, preterm labor, growth retardation, and the reduction of head circumference in infants (Mulder et al. 2002).

Insight into epigenetics is a part of my daily work of carving out memories (Brock 2017). The science of memory and epigenetics is concerned with how mundane and ordinary things are perceived and how they influence us (Kida 2014; Candau 2010). Our daily actions provide the basis of these sciences, and every movement repeated by mothers becomes embedded in memories and becomes a transgenerational conductor (Anderson 2015a; Christie and Pim 2012; Ward 2008). Essentially, a mother's experiences can influence epigenetic processes and fine-tune gene expression in the child toward the best possible thriving mechanisms (Ollikainen et al. 2010).

Research has shown that maternal fright and trauma can cause transgenerational epigenetic changes (Clemmons 2000; Jablonka and Lamb 2005; de Mendelssohn 2008) and that traumatic experiences can be passed down through our DNA (deMause 2006; Carey 2013). The mother's memories and life experiences are remembered by the children and can lead to tragic consequences in their developing brains and bodies. In other words, the wars and violence perpetrated onto the mother and the environment are virally penetrating.

The life experiences and memories of our ancestors, mothers, and grandmothers can change our gene expression, and by the same biological mechanism, maternal fright propagates an assortment of ills. According to Eric Kandel's (2007) work on the neurobiology of memory, new memories are layered over the original ones (see also Eichenbaum and Fortin 2009). Research has noted that the same process plays a role in passing down genetic diseases and programming, such as Rett syndrome and severe autism.

This continues to be observed by the South Slavic women survivors after a century of wars. Since the life experiences of grandmothers become the lived memories of grandchildren, what we have is an epigenetic process that concentrates in the preconception stages of the mother's and father's life experiences, and perinatal, gestational, and early childhood development (Anderson 2015a; Burton et al. 2010).

MATERNAL FRIGHT CHANGES CIRCADIAN RHYTHMS

Women who are war survivors often reported that their circadian rhythms were disrupted and unable to return to an adaptive state. These women also reported an inheritance of maternal fright (Christie and Pim 2012; Anderson 2015a). Somehow, through their oral memory traditions, that involves an interaction of the science of rituals with bioneurological and epigenetic processes, the women survivors understood their natural circadian rhythms can be maintained and can even restore health, thus eradicating maternal fright.

More importantly, the female tacit knowledge, evolving over thousands of years, appears to depend on the rhythm and synchronization of our biological clock, which is universally based on light and dark cycles. Circadian misalignment disrupts our physiological rhythms, wreaking havoc on our bodies and health, resulting in conditions such as diabetes, obesity, and heart problems, as well as the epigenetic processes that result in maternal fright (Laber-Warren 2015, 33).

ORAL MEMORY TRADITIONS ARE CLOSELY INTERTWINED BIOLOGICAL RHYTHMS

What I have observed and researched with regard to healing women's trauma are the oral memory traditions, which are found to be in sync with maternal biological rhythms (Hannon and Johnson 2005; Anderson 2014a). The development of culture's cradle is the semiosphere where the emergence of life consists of encircling flesh membranes in its self-organizing states. We are talking about the storied developmental perinatal stages—female biology twined with nature (Sebeok 2001).

Sinc I consider the oral memory traditions to be the translation of neural codes defining the self-organizing states producing iconic epigenetic memory narratives, stories, and mythologies, inclusive of female biology and the diversity of nature. The oral memory practices are a result, loaded with ballads, chants, and dances to rituals of daily life practices (Kull and Velmezova 2019; Roesler 2012).

Carl Jung's great works on archetypes and the symbolic and his statement that culture is a part of man's nature is somewhat accurate (Jung and von Franz 1968). What is not included in Jung's statement is the reality that culture is rooted in female biology and her nature (Mies 1998; Tannen 2014).

The maternal biological rhythms form oral memory traditions via repetitive life practices and life experiences. In essence, oral memory traditions preserve the knowledge of biological processes and female memories of conception, pregnancy, and birth without written manuals, transgenerationally layered membranes of culture. These traditions are what I refer to as female tacit knowledge and what biosemioticans recognize as "knowledge is then fed into the present and may, in that way, also alter the past is known to human beings" (Wheeler 2006b, 9; Gifford 2010). The structure of maternal biological rhythms and processes entail many daily processes from menstruation to menopause (Bledsoe and Banja 2002; Bateson 2001), but none are as critical to this book as maternal fright and the focus on perinatal stages.

Moreover, I noted how oral memory traditions house an archetypal constellation of life experiences, and concepts of epigenetic propensities and neuroscience provide venues for clarifying how female social collectives are distinct from the assemblies of traumatized individuals (Anderson 2014a; 2015a). It is the female social collectives, the biological roots of nature that are represented in the oral memory traditions practices—a group culture that is vastly different from isolated traumatized individuals (Freudenburg and Jones 1991).

Yet, the female social collective harbingers of culture and of oral memory traditions are treated as harmless folklore, not worthy of science or governing entities (Giesen 2004; Grünberg 2009). In this context, the South Slavic female social collectives are to proclaim a nonpolitical status so as not to offend the men and that powers that be, despite the reality that what is political is personal for women evidenced with a century of war and war crimes against her. Yet, "women around the world at every sociopolitical level find themselves under-represented in parliament and far removed from decision-making levels. While the political playing field in each country has its own particular characteristics, one feature remains common to all: it is uneven and not conducive to women's participation. Throughout the world women face obstacles to their participation in politics" (Thanikodi and Sugirtha 2007, 589).

Also related to this is the controversial inheritance of personality traits, temperament behavioral genetics, and studies of the interactions of genes and the environment, showing that there is a correlation to traditional oral memory practices. This is a science of rituals with symbols, motifs, and scripts found in artifacts and pottery, and is currently easily identified in the South Slavic embroidery, kilim-rugs, and daily life practices (Steinberg et al. 2010). Before, the alphabet and written words, preliterate cultures used repetition to pass down storied instructions into memory. According to the linguist and independent scholar Harald Haarmann (1997), "European literacy in the pre-alphabetic context is one pattern in which various aspects of cultural continuity over a period of several millennia can be observed" (119).

Given the indivisible world of interrelationships, I cannot avoid the maternal uterine environment, which is rarely included in research. A compelling concept for me is that the fetus in the womb is vulnerable to the mother's natural rhythms of temperature, food/nutrition, and melatonin. For example, maternal melatonin is one of the few hormones that remains in its chemical state without being altered in the blood, and that synchronizes the fetus's rhythms to those of the mother, producing the semiosphere (Serón-Ferré et al. 2012; Kull and Velmezova 2019).

The mother's daily life, a rhythmic circadian semiosphere, has the fetus in the womb vulnerable to the mother's natural rhythms of temperature, food/nutrition, and melatonin, highlighted in times of violence and wars. The women survivors of war crimes in the aftermath of the Balkan War knew this, and the kolo of mothers and grandmothers worked to ensure that the best possible daily life and nutritional needs were provided (Anderson 2015b).

The absorbing question that arises with the women war survivors is how they knew this and understand the complexity of their female biology. A study on gestation and the close relationship between mother and the fetus reports,

> by living inside the maternal compartment, the fetus is inevitably exposed to rhythms of the maternal internal milieu such as temperature; rhythms originated

> by maternal food intake and maternal melatonin, one of the few maternal hormones that cross the placenta unaltered. This may also extend to the developing circadian system. We propose that the fetal suprachiasmatic nucleus (SCN) of the hypothalamus and fetal organs are peripheral maternal circadian oscillators, entrained by different maternal signals. (Serón-Ferré et al. 2012, 68)

However, the term "maternal compartment," as opposed to the womb, shows the inherent male bias that can account for the lack of perinatal and fetal female biology studies and knowledge in the science (Perez 2021).

By thriving in the uterine environment, the fetus develops and eventually transitions into being a thriving newborn, a member of a future generation. Without maternal fright, the uterine environment returns to a state of equilibrium "since biology can tell us anything about culture" (Wheeler 2006b, 22). Culture rooted in biology is geared toward coevolution of an adaptive culture and society.

What is affected are the evolving and healing practices of the South Slavic women's oral memory traditions, prompted by the uterine environment orchestrated in complex biological systems, ecologies, and into human societies via the nature of agency.

Maternal/female tacit knowledge is based in the body, and female experiential knowledge is based in the oral memory traditions and is associated with the fractal geometry of complex systems (Polanyi 1966). Fractal geometry, in recent research, has shown the vast natural creative forms from coastlines and trees to the body, blood, brain, and lungs (Briggs and Peat 1989, 90–91). For example, medical science when studying the fetal brain uses the fractal dimension to measure the increases in vessel calibers. The most rapid growth in fractal dimension is in the sixth and seventh month of gestation, and is known as an effective tool to measure the structures of the brain vessels (Kedzia et al., 2002).

Maternal/Female tacit knowledge, a capacity to self-organize (autopoiesis—focus in hereditary transfers) into natural knowledge, has existed since prehistoric times and is embedded in female collective memory recorded in our gene expression (Wheeler 2006b; Polanyi 1966; von Bertalanffy 1968). Prehistorically, that maternal tacit knowledge from millennia of her life experiences led to the development of oral memory practices, before the reign of wars and violence, five thousand years ago (Wheeler 2006b; Eisler 1991).

What is so resilient and resourceful within the South Slavic oral memory traditions is that they are easily perpetuated throughout the generations, despite the numerous wars, conquests, or other formidable obstacles (Anderson 2014a; Christie and Pim 2012). Given that culture is created through women and their biological processes, producing oral memory traditions and rituals aligned with our neurobiology and perinatal and natal spheres, women, and in this case, South Slavic women, are an invaluable resource with the capacity to eradicate transgenerational trauma.

An oral memory tradition, the kolo, to be in a circle or a folk round dance, is a practice that mirrors the biological rhythms and entrainment for our circadian system to synchronize, not just the mother and fetus, but also the social collective that Porges (2007) calls social engagement in the dance or circle. In Belgrade Serbia, kolo dancing is held in Avala Park with hundreds participating to this day (Boxell 2019). With the South Slavic and Bosnian women survivors of war crimes and war, the kolo was employed as the beginning of healing.

Since maternal biological rhythms hold similar patterns to fetal circadian rhythms, it evokes emotional states, as noted in studies. I posit that the maternal circadian rhythms are essential for the developmental fetal brain functions (Reppert and Schwartz 1984). Given that the fetus responds to cues from the maternal signals, and that the fetal circadian rhythm is entrained with the mothers,' conceptually the arrangement of the mother and uterine environment disposes a temporal order during fetal life (Serón-Ferré et al. 2012).

The oral memory traditions and practices are in synchrony with the maternal circadian cycles by incorporating music-chants, song, instruments, dance, and domestic life to self-sustainability (Anderson 2016).

To eradicate maternal fright, the Bosnian women survivors relied on their oral memory traditions and practices. However, when the South Slavic women war crimes and war survivors had nothing, enduring their refugee status and loss of safety after a century of wars, they discovered that their capacity they had everything; their South Slavic culture and oral memory traditions embedded with female tacit maternal knowledge.

With their female tacit maternal knowledge, these women understood that "life of a complex system is not reducible to its constituent parts" (the whole is greater than its parts) (Wheeler 2006b, 53). The small domestic life acts are highly influenced and sensitive to the environment and are outcomes of healing trauma impacts practices (Anderson 2014a; Christie and Pim 2012; Polanyi 1962).

Chapter 5

Female Social Justice

Oral Memory Traditions Kolo

The purpose of holocaust museums is to immerse participants in the past events of genocide and of war crimes (Alexander 2012). The process of physically constructing the museums is akin to the construction of the South Slavic females' oral memory traditions. For example, the creation of physical structures to memorialize and reexperience the Holocaust in museums is a process that unfolds similarly for the South Slavic oral memory traditions created by the female war crimes and war survivors (J. E. Young 1993). In fact, the South Slavic oral memory traditions, and global oral memory traditions are visible when people have nothing.

However, the women's creation of the oral memories does not have a purpose to promote hatred in response to the holocaustic events, as might be said of the museums due to the sway and misinformation found in social media that the Holocaust never happened (Germain 2022). Rather, women's abilities to heal from the events are a form of social justice that can be passed down through the generations. Justice is portrayed in the women's collective participation in the somatic release of the folk round dances known in Serbo-Croatian as the kolo, meaning "to be in a circle" and representing daily life practices that range from a collective trauma healing to social justice (Christie and Pim 2012).

The Mesolithic kolo enacted is a living museum of ancestors' life experiences erected into the present moment (Ilieva and Shturbanova 1997). Many elder women survivors of war crimes and war would organize and push for a celebration ritual with dance, music, and food whenever divides and high tension were occurring in the community, threatening to explode into violence or wars (Kolo Sumcjja Women (KSW) War Crimes and War Survivors 2000–2022). Interestingly, many elder women would often point out that it is not easy to kill someone you danced or sat in a circle in the kolo with (KSW 2000–2022).

With many returns to Novi Travnik, Bosnia, it was hailed with press conferences and at the local level, the women war crimes, either with live music or with the ancient cassette tape of kolo dances, orchestrated a somatic polyvagal movement that is a "vagal brake which can promote transitory mobilization and the expression of sympathetic tone without requiring sympathetic or adrenal activities" (Porges 2011, 158). With the sympathetic fright/flight found in response to danger, and living in the aftermath of the Balkan War, the trauma impacts are prolonged adrenaline survival responses that biologically will shut down metabolic processes and blood flow to the stomach and to parts of brain (Porges 2011, 159).

With the inclusion of the Mesolithic kolo dances and circles, the women war crimes and war survivors were attuned to the need for the vagal brake on the sympathetic fright/flight. At the same time, the kolo, a living museum collective is the "human matrix carrying the encoded story of our race, back to its very genesis. All those alive today have been entrusted to hold this living record and chosen by evolution to update and renew it into a new tomorrow" (Hubl 2020, 11).

The array of organically self-sustainabity, with food grown from their own balconies or rented plots of land, Bosnian Muslim food to Croatian and Serbian, is a bioculinary, life/culinary medicinal practice, and is a living agrarian and food science museum—the backdrop at the kolo dances and circles (Anderson 2012a). Certainly, the blood flow resumed to the stomach and every bite strikes deep with meaning and herstory over history. Gracefully, the kolo meanders from culture to biology to recipes, embracing the importance of memory. It is savored, reexperienced with both genetic and tacit knowledge learned, via daily life (Anderson 2012a).

Given, the women war crimes and war survivors have endured a century of wars and genocide, the three major wars only strengthened their oral memory traditions somatically. But the oral memory tradition, embedded in the somatic psychological practice of the kolo, likened to life and death, is a matter of surviving or thriving, and have enhanced the healing of the South Slavic women (thriving) or have disappeared as a result of the intense trauma (surviving) (Anderson 2012a; 2012b).

For example, many of the women war crimes and war survivors report they do not want to remember or repeat what happened to them, and a few have amnesia (KSW 2000–2022). Additionally, the women war crimes and war survivors report that their memories that they have experienced, and that of their children, have been omitted, ensuring that that they do not exist, as if the war crimes and war events never happened (Anderson 2015b).

The issue for the women war crimes and war survivors is the reality that their male relatives whether, Croat, Bosnijak-Muslim, or Serb, were the perpetrators (KSW 2000–2022; Anderson 2015a; 2015b).

Poring through many research essays/data, journal papers, and books that can point to the tacit knowing and situations where I witnessed self-healing trauma, it is very rare that the subject is contained in the psychological science field. Antonio Damasio (2018) writes "the abundant recall of related memories sustains and amplifies suffering [pain and memories of suffering]. Memory helps project the situation into the imagined future and lets us envision the consequences" (11; see also Damasio 2010).

In my "kolo-informed trauma care," the women survivors of war crimes and war do not leave it at the point of imaging a future (Anderson 2015a). What I have witnessed, not just in the Balkans but across the globe, is the point where movement, oral memory traditions—dance, song, music or gathering in a social collective—moves from suffering and pain memories into the present moment of healing and a reauthoring of their lives, thus families and communities.

What I know to be true is found in Damasio's work. In his book *Self Comes to Mind: Constructing the Conscious Brain*, Damasio (2010) explained that "high levels of emotion signal the hippocampus to store memories long-term; unless an event is of great threat, danger or terror, the hippocampus ignores it. The neurological reasoning necessary for editing out what is not imperative to survival and preserving what is recorded long-term in the brain memory allows for the most significant long-term memories to consist of higher cognitive processes" (112).

For example, women's eradication of oral memory traditions, such as the artifacts from mass graves, indicates a grave dismissal of their grieving and their mourning process (Steinmaurer et al. 2021; Bentz et al. 2013). The case in point is the Srebrenica women war crimes survivors who were reeling with the September 2009 Yugoslav War Crimes Tribunal's decision to destroy any artifacts from the mass graves of their male relatives (Horsthuis 2019; Deasy and Halimovic 2009). The cold logic and masculine dominion over the war crimes survivors, mostly women and widows, has been and will continue to be a status quo that adds insult to injury to keep post-traumatic stress disorder (PTSD) in heightened conditioning (Cockburn 2013).

Cynthia Cockburn (2013) determined "women have recently intervened internationally to argue that if peace is to be [more] than a mere cessation of hostilities, 'security' must be redefined to mean the satisfaction of human needs, including comprehensive safety for women. Women's peace movements worldwide are theorizing that gender power relations are significant among the cause of war and transformative change in how we 'live' gender can be a significant resource for peace" (433).

Female social justice and South Slavic female humanities oral memory traditions have mortuary images and oral memory traditions that are as powerful as the four-thousand-year-old artifacts that are strewn about in the former

Yugoslav regions. The social memory is found in the simple watch locates and in localizes images of the past, in specific places and spaces of their lives. The images of memory, although fragmentary and provisional, heal and continue the archeomythological storytelling of the cataclysmic violence that have scared their lives. The bottom line is that the Srebrenica widows and mothers instruction intensified learning whenever trauma appears in their lives.

The South Slavic women war crimes and war survivors in their regional excursions and in kolo circles worked with the mothers and supported their outcries. Through their kolo circles, a wide network was woven, transcending not just international borders but also the victim role of women war crimes and war survivors (KSW 2000–2022).

The Radio Free Europe article of an interview with a mother, Subasic, reported "that a number of mothers who lost children 'don't have photographs of them,'" explaining that "if you don't have a mezar [a Muslim grave], if you don't have photographs if you don't have anything that belonged to that person, it's like the person never existed. Those things put us in a position to prove that we did have our children" (Deasy and Halimovic 2009).

Wanting to forget—amnesia due to the war crimes and war memories—can have devastating consequences. Being immigrants or refugees and fleeing to safety when there is no safe place and where the denial and repression of memories to include one's cultural oral memory recycles into a ceaseless survival mechanism, thus easily dropped into the victim role (Oxfam International 2023; Porges 2007).

While comparisons may be made by looking at mass shootings, especially in the United State and that are on the increase, my focus is specifically on the Balkan War refugees and immigrants. The diaspora and refugee status that the women war crimes and war survivors endure, indicate that the impact of their trauma is not healed, due in part to not having their oral memory traditions and a lack of mental health services (B. Allen 1996). On February 15, 2007, the media reported on the Bosnian-born teen, Sulejman Talovic, aged eighteen years. Talovico killed five people and wounded four others in a shooting spree at a US shopping mall (CBS News 2007). Not long after the shooting spree, the women survivors of war crimes and war contacted me to request that I call the mother, whom they knew.

At the age of three years old, Talovic survived bombs, snipers, and knowing the fate of eight thousand other Muslims males, who were massacred in 1995 at Srebrenica. Instead, Talovic was shot to death by Utah police after his murdering rampage in Salt Lake City. The CBS/AP article quoted the following from relatives: "I saw it on TV, and I heard a brave policeman killed the shooter. Not in my wildest dreams could I have presumed Sulejman killed those people. When I heard his name, I fell from the sofa" said Redzo Talovic, a fifty-nine-year-old cousin of the gunman. "What got into him? This is what we are all asking ourselves. We are all in shock" (CBS News 2007).

Globally accepted and patriarchally institutionalized is the blame and shame behind Redzo Talovic' s shock, implying that he and his family did not see it or that they did nothing to prevent it, despite dealing with their survivorship. Since society glorifies those who fight, accept the fright/flight while attaching shame and the immobilization—not doing anything—the focus needs to be on the person's response and not to the traumatic event. For Talovic, the mass gun shooter's adverse childhood experiences—on a scale that vastly accumulates and thus increases the probability of suicide, addiction, and psychiatric disorders and psychoses later into adulthood—are neglected (Anthony 2019).

According to an interview by Andrew Anthony (2019) with Porges,

> Much of our society defines trauma by the event when the real critical issue is the individual's reaction. By not accepting that, we end up saying: "If I can survive this and do well, why can't you?" So, we start blaming the survivors again. The point that we have to understand is that when a person has a reaction or response to trauma, the body interprets the traumatic event as a life threat. There's a massive retuning of how the nervous system works, how it regulates underlying physiological systems that impact social behavior, psychological experiences, and also on physical outcomes. (Anthony 2019)

Repression of trauma memories, especially with those who experienced violence, living in a war zone at a young nonverbal age is prime for transgenerational trauma. There are no words for what is witnessed or experienced. Hence, there were no signs that the eighteen-year-old was in trouble and having a difficult time adjusting to Utah as well as the high school bullying. Since the deeply repressed memories are buried, trauma has us responding as victims with steel-reinforced denial (Otgaar et al. 2021). Srebrenica war widows and their families waited for decades, thinking their sons, husbands, brothers, and uncles were just missing. The Srebrenica widows remarked on how missing for years is as if their relatives never existed, therefore, cannot be a genocide trauma memory or mass murder victims.

In part, the Srebrenica war crimes survivors and the Bosnian women war survivors evoked survival mechanisms neurobiologically to "repress or push traumatic memories aside, allowing a person to cope and move forward" (Jones 2021; Kandel 2007).

Denial meant not speaking of the reality, let alone facing it. I asked the women war crimes and war survivors and Srebrenica war widows why there were one hundred years of war in their backyards and homes. The women war crimes and war survivors responded in waves of blame, attesting the hierarchal property of our language and communications today as, "They came and took our sons, husbands, and uncles away" (KSW 2000–2022).

But who are, "They?" The Srebrenica war widows vehemently shouted, "the Serbs." The Novi Travnik/Kolo Sumejja women said, "the Croats." Still ignited with an intense curiosity and a compelling need to understand who "they" were, was due to the women war crimes and war survivors being very comfortable with the term "they."

When I inquired where their sons and husbands or fathers were during the conflict, mostost were fighting somewhere else.

Given that their husbands, brothers, and sons—along with their fathers—killed other people over there had the women survivors of war crimes and war at first, erupting in rage. However, the question that needed to be asked was "do those women call their beloved and family, 'they?'" (KSW 2000–2022).

What was a significant and obvious pattern in their response was that "they" are our husbands, sons, and uncles. Understanding the term "they" ignited a shocking clarity, since the Srebrenica war crimes widows and Novi Travnik-Vitez women war crimes and war survivors were defending their missing but describing the slaughtered male relatives as "good boys and men." The reality is that their male relatives, also like the women, are victims, no matter what side they belonged to in the war.

The women war crimes and war survivors understood they are not to be blamed nor shamed. Nor are their male relatives, or the men and women on the other sides of war, to feel the brunt of blame.

The loss of the Slavic kolo, the circle, the Slavic Moist Mother Earth cultural reverence in every part of their lives appeared to be irrevocably lost in their transgenerational trauma. What insight was had by the women war crimes and war survivors of the "land of they" was the ever-looming patriarchal element that institutionalizes strife and divisions. Hiding the reality that men are perpetrators, and the good men are bystanders, either silent victim or a part of their male entitlement and power over play a major role in "land of they," perpetuating transgenerational trauma thus eradicating adaptive cultural social responses.

As an outsider and Serbian American whose father who had no formal education and was a World War II partisan with Yugoslav's King Peter and General Mihailovic, the women war crimes and war survivors accepted me and my informed trauma work. However, at the start of the clinical informed trauma treatments, upon hearing my lineage, the women war survivors were rageful, ensuing a rampage of "they did this to them" in their responses (KSW 2000–2022).

Then, the elder women asked me why I came and keep returning. I pointed out the loss of the South Slavic and Slavic culture and social behaviors and the repression of memory, my mother's silence, a World War II Jasenovac concentration camp survivor (Anderson 2015a). My response was I did not want my children or my grandchildren to have life experiences of my father and mother, and to realize that there is no way they did this, it is we who did this.

The recognition of our participation, either as a victim or perpetrator, bystander though extremely painful, the shadow of transgenerational trauma is powerful enough to dismiss the cultural collective healing of transgenerational trauma. The informed trauma session, land of they, with the women war survivors had a grandmother whose children and grandchildren are flung across the globe; it is a diaspora so cutting to the South Slavic matrilineal culture that she responded with one sentence: "I raised my children to hate" (KSW 2000–2022).

Hauntingly like Talovic' s relatives and mother, who stated he was such a good boy after the Utah shooting spree, adaptive cultural memory is evidently replaced by trauma induced by violence, a contagious viral transgenerational trauma.

Warping the oral memories, intergenerational trauma etched in after one hundred years of war, Talovic carried the legacies of his fathers and their fathers before him. He would pay for the sins of the fathers as he languished in trauma striving to be the "good patriarchal son." He suffered through bullying and domestic violence issues—both psychic and physical but called "culture" and "this is the way it is."

The young man, just on the brink of his entire life, has been expunged from our memories through our denial and inaction on healing intergenerational trauma by stationing mothers/females onto one of the lowest rungs of the proverbial ladder. The hierarchal-patriarchal life taking judgments (blame/shame), the transgenerational trauma shadow dismisses matrilineal cultural memory practices sealing the secondary citizenship status for women and children via blaming and shaming them (Anderson 2015a). Yet, it is mothers who raise our sons and daughters precisely from the valueless assignment.

But statistics are so overwhelmingly obvious and shocking. It is men who account for 90 percent of the perpetrators of violent crimes, and in wars, slaughter each other (Perez 2021). It is androcide, the systematic killing of men, boys, or males, who globally constitute 79 percent of nonconflict wars homicides and direct-conflict war deaths (Gibbons 2013; Ormhaug et al. 2009). The Srebrenica androcide of male relatives during the Balkan War is an example. An estimated 100,000 people were killed in the Balkan War, and 80 percent were Bosnijak-Muslims, with an estimate of 8,000 to 10,000 Bosnian males from Srebrenica becoming the largest massacre in Europe since the Holocaust (United States Holocaust Memorial Museum 2013).

The reality is that women are in denial about these statistics, given it is too horrific to comprehend thus unspeakable. What women do comprehend is their sense of powerlessness. That denial halts any chance of evolutionary memory, the healing of collective trauma, and serves to only repeats an endless addictive cycle intergenerationally (Anderson 2015b; Njaka and Peacock 2021). What is meant by evolutionary memory is a controversial quantum psychology, and in philosophy, the theory of retrocausality that influences the present or the future to change the past (Hubl 2020, 7).

According to Joanna Hubl (2020) what is human sociability and matrilineal cultural behaviors and brings about retrocausality opens to the "the truth of our interrelation and interdependence . . . our unhealed cultural history. We can connect and cohere. We discover ourselves as a new kind of being distinctly individual, yet profoundly collective" (195).

Does women's plight and violence toward women hold men accountable? Does the enforced silence of women and mothers, who conform to become their father's daughter and the patriarch's esteemed mother, offer up their children for future generations? How do we treat newcomers and travelers to our land? Do we say, like the Africans, "Welcome back."

Due to these transgenerational trauma impacts, the women war survivors reported that they do not have the money to travel to Sarajevo, Bosnia and Hercegovina, and why would they want to, since there is no need, and because no women's memories narratives are included. Pointing to the Yugoslav Tribunal adjudicating that the war crimes that occurred in Vitez on April 16, 1993, never happened thus their war crimes and war memories are eradicated. One elder war survivor stated, "now they have us killing ourselves" (KSW 2000–2022).

Daniel Schacter (1997), a Harvard psychologist, in his studies of neuroimaging, backs up what the Slavs have practiced in their mythic Mesolithic narratives; he and his colleagues discovered that the same brain circuits are involved in both remembering events and imagining, thus creating adaptive events.

Other studies have suggested that amnesia is basically the loss of one's ability to imagine or to have an imagination, which impacts their visions for a future since they cannot imagine or visualize creative acts (Kandel 2006). Hence, modern-day museums are central to culture wars, mostly toward fabulous funding and urban locations those memorializing men and the patriotism of war heroes to male inventors, basically not relevant since memory and life experiences of ancestors are not brought forward to the present moment or inclusive in nature. Nicholas Thomas (2019), in *Apollo* magazine, notes "museums therefore needed to diversify audiences, and not only increase numbers but engage 'hard to reach' communities, attracting those who had not previously visited them. The challenge has had wide-ranging implications for curatorial work and programming: museums have needed to be seen as inviting, inclusive and 'relevant.'"

In relation to South Slavic oral memory traditions, the women's visions for a future may be jeopardized if they cannot imagine or visualize the form of a future nonkilling culture with nonviolent cultural memories. If the South Slavic oral memory traditions have not been lost to amnesia, the memories have recorded the practices experienced by ancestors for thousands of generations, including those that are tainted by violence and have endured.

Since this population of female victims has been neglected in terms of research on their experiences of war trauma and South Slavic oral memory traditions, it remains unclear how their traumatic experiences may have affected their collective memory practices (Herman 1992; Knight 2002; Knight et al. 1995; Mertus 2000; Schulz 2005). There are at least three obstacles to address when considering the effects of trauma on the this population: (1) the cultural taboos of being Muslim and of being Bosnian; (2) the marginal and invisible status of females worldwide, resulting in studies having largely ignored the plight of women in war, genocide, and female oral memory traditions; and (3) the fact that women, being largely invisible, comprise most of the war's collateral damage statistics (Campbell 2002; Mertus 2000; Totten 2009; Vlachovà and Biason 2004). These obstacles must be considered in relation to the women's use of oral memory traditions in hopes of better understanding and of improving the lives of these women.

THE IMPACT OF WAR ON CULTURAL TRADITIONS

Violent conflicts and wars target the homes of thousands of civilians, with a clear example being present in the South Slavic war crimes and war survivors. Adam Roberts (1999) documented what is called "collateral damage" in Kosovo. As of March 1999, Roberts estimated there were 260,000 internally displaced persons (IDP) and at least 100,000 refugees and asylum seekers in the region. The most comprehensive example of collateral damage is provided by the Humanitarianism and War Project by Julie A. Mertus (2000). Mertus estimated the number of displaced persons and refugees to include 75 percent to 80 percent war-imperiled women and their children who have been fleeing or have been forcibly removed from their homes. Given this significant portion of the population, the current research focuses on the South Slavic Muslim female survivors who have endured the collateral damage imposed by the Balkan War.

When women and children are displaced from their regions of origin, their cultural memory traditions are at risk of being lost. Intangible heritage and cultural memory traditions and practices include pieces of information that represent meaning and energy for a group of people (Johnson and Grand 1998; Siegel 2008). Neuroscientists understand how the brain, our neurological network, is shaped by information and by energy (Rossi 2002; Siegel 2008).

With recent findings in neuroscience, we are beginning to understand how ethnic and cultural traditions tie into our neurological and biological processes (Hanson and Mendius 2009). By studying the South Slavic females' intangible heritage and cultural memory traditions, a symbolic logic (Knight 1987), we can better understand the collective component in which their oral memory tradition practices are embedded in their culture, which will inform somatic psychological practices. However, the critical underlying factor to focus on these aspects of intangible heritage, or the daily living of these women, is to first recognize how violent conflicts, wars, and even natural disasters impact females in many vulnerable areas of daily life (Alexander et al. 2004; Roberts 1999).

ORAL MEMORY TRADITIONS AND WORLD WAR II

In World War II, concentration camps were used for the mass killings of Jews, Gypsies, Muslims, and Serbs; these atrocities were repeated in the Balkan War rape camps (Lifton 2000; Stiglmayer 1993). The lack of empirical reference to the South Slavic war crimes in historical accounts of wartime affairs follows suit in the lack of research on the impact of trauma on oral memory traditions. The World War II sterilization methods enforced by the Nazis targeted the most vulnerable population: women. Given that women create culture privileged by their female biology, oral memory traditions are body centered. For example, the term "City of Mothers" was used to describe Carl Clauberg's (1898–1957) institution for sterility and reproduction, aiming for a new enhanced race so that the destruction of the womb is in actuality the destruction of the female oral memory traditions (Kaupen-Haas 1988).

Ignoring women and their bodies is not particularly unusual for holocaustic trauma research. A review of the literature on the Jewish Holocaust of World War II included little data on women (United States Holocaust Memorial Museum 2011). Although Emanuel Ringelblum (1900–1944) broached the topic of how female holocaustic experiences were neglected after World War II, it was only recently that female trauma specific to sex and reproduction has been explored, while relatively little research has studied female oral memory traditions as a somatic psychological practice (as cited in Totten 2009, 4). Graça Macel reported on the impacts of war on women's daily lives, including the harmful consequences of mass rapes and struggles in postconflict periods (as cited in Totten 2009, 83–107). Golie G. Jansen (2006) pointed out that gender inequality may be more pronounced during conflicts, presenting greater impact upon females' health and mental health since women are the most vulnerable.

Likewise, Mertus (2000) used a feminist perspective to point out that gender-based violence is a calculated methodology during war, used to force entire populations to flee. These studies, however, ignore the impact of this trauma upon oral memory traditions (Zajicek and Calasanti 1998; Perez 2021; Mertus 2000; Olujic 1998; Totten 2009).

ORAL MEMORY TRADITIONS AND RECENT WARS

Recent clinical studies began a focused approach to investigate the effects of trauma on menstruation. Mary Ellen Doherty and Elizabeth Scannell-Desch (2012) conducted research on women's health and experiences during deployment to the Iraq and Afghanistan War from 2003 to 2010. The population focused on nurses, due to their existing medical knowledge. More importantly, the study revolved around women's daily lives in a combat situation. In considering war-related violence against women, menstruation was found to be affected by both physical and psychological trauma.

Maria B. Olujic (1998) reported that female bodies, specifically their sexuality and reproductive processes, are manipulated as weapons of war. The RAM plan, first developed in 1991 by Serbian forces, is the first document of planned genocide and terrorizing of Muslim females with rape camps (Allen 1996). Beverly Allen's (1996) book *Rape Warfare: The Hidden Genocide in Bosnia-Herzegovina and Croatia*, she notes: "a variation of the RAM Plan, written by the army's special services, including . . . experts in psychological warfare" (57). The author offers a chilling sociological rationale for the tactics of ethnic cleansing:

> Our analysis of the behavior of the Muslim communities demonstrates that the morale, will, and bellicose nature of their groups can be undermined *only if we aim our action at the point where the religious and social structure is most fragile. We refer to the women, especially adolescents, and to the children.* Decisive intervention on these social figures would spread confusion . . . , thus causing first of all fear and then panic, leading to a probable retreat from the territories involved in war activity. (Allen 1996, location 899)

It is estimated that anywhere between 20,000 to 50,000 South Slavic females, mostly targeted female Muslims, were raped during the Balkan War from 1991 through 1994 (Mertus 2000; Stiglmayer 1993). What is interesting to note is that the ethnic and cultural aspect of South Slavic women's capacity to bear children is taken by a patriarchal rule to beget sons (Anderson 2015a).

In Sara Meger's (2011) report, which focused on violence against women in the Democratic Republic of the Congo, the author described the policies across the globe, "that construct sexual violence as an effective and strategic weapon of war. Genocidal rape has been used throughout history to humiliate defeated groups and to sully the bloodlines of the 'enemy'" (as cited in Allen 1996, location 60). The absence of theory, as related to the gynocidal rape and trauma impacts, in examining female somatic processes and the interrelationships of conceiving and preserving oral memory traditions are seldom noted (Campbell 2002; J. Fisher 2010; Knight, 1987).

Yet, the rape camps, and the fact that 75 percent to 80 percent of global refugees are women, have the creators of culture—women—unable to partake in domestic daily practices, a part of oral memory traditions, and they struggle to heal and deal with severe trauma as a result (Fisher and Ogden 2009; Mertus 2000).

A significant factor about the genocidal rape camps was the nature of the captors in the former Yugoslavia region. The men understood female biological processes in addition to knowing how potent South Slavic females' oral memory traditions perpetuate a nonkilling culture (Bahtijaragic and Pim 2015). The rape camp perpetrators instituted rape camps to increase the odds of pregnancies for female prisoners, adding to the women's further humiliation (Allen 1996; Mertus 2000; Stiglmayer 1993).

But something more was occurring at a deeper cultural tissue. In the Balkan War, rape camps were not just targeting younger women, but also older women who had education and who were highly regarded, resulting in an impact of up to three generations of female caregivers (Allen 1996; Mertus 2000; Olujic 1998). Thus, when studying the impact of trauma on oral memory traditions, it will be necessary to consider the age of the women to determine how the levels of trauma are healed or not attended to, through the female oral memory traditions.

As actors in a multivariant drama series of episodic violence and war events, the women must reconsider their direct connections to ancestors in the remembered past or with a vague mythological antiquity, offering reinterpretations for recovery purposes (International Criminal Tribunal for the former Yugoslavia [ICTY] 1995). For example, one Ahmica grandmother continues to use the oven in which her grandchild was baked to death on April 16, 1994, known as the day of Ahmica war crimes.

The woman has overwritten the terrible memory through the daily use of her oven, changing and eventually healing the neurological process of memory while maintaining a mythic sorrowful narrative of her grandchild. The human geography, the space and place of her wood-burning stove, once evoked a genocidal memory of bitterness, but with the daily use of the stove, her fragrant bread-making, and the preparation of cultural dishes have embraced the memorial of her grandchild (Anderson 2012a or 2012b).

For women like the South Slavic grandmother, the presence of *signs* and iconic representations serve as notices to the Ahmica community to make meaning after the onslaught on the domestic realm. The onslaught most significantly impacted women from middle age to the elderly, who held the rich daily ceremonies of coffee and cup readings along with being in a circle together and the Kolo round dancing (Christie and Pim 2012). During the twenty-plus-year period of my engagements with the women, the setting of the environment of South Slavic mythic narratives and oral traditions often commenced with the gathering of women (Anderson 2012a or 2012b).

The Ahmica women war crimes survivors met with the author by coming together in the largest home. Sitting on the floor with handmade kilims while coffee was served on large silver platters, the sharing of the women's survival stories commenced. They thrived on iconic representations of loved ones, such as the woman who returned home only to die from cancer a few months later.

The storyline seized and gained ground when the recounts of the woman proliferated on her disenfranchised status as a displaced person. Her displaced status was ultimately hinged on being able to die gracefully in her bed in the only home she ever knew. Her home became the flag, or the icon, at which the women pointed to her home and referred to her saga. At times, the surviving community of women planted flowers at the woman's home after her death to tend to and nurture the home and the woman all at the same time. In this way, the Ahmica women's seasonal and daily acts are converted symbolically through the mythic narrative process.

ORAL MEMORY TRADITIONS, BIOLOGICAL, AND NEUROLOGICAL PROCESSES

In reviewing the literature, it is necessary to consider the fields of biology, neuroscience, and somatic psychology to distinguish possible relationships between surviving war and holocaust and South Slavic oral memory traditions (Christie and Pim 2012; Fisher and Ogden 2009; Olujic 1998). Placing women and their oral memory traditions at the center of the research allows a fuller examination of variability in the traumatized women's experiences, highlighting how their basic biological practices have been affected by the trauma (Anderson 2012a or 2012b; Christie and Pim 2012; Campbell 2002; Totten 2009).

Jamie L. Rhudy and Emily J. Bartley (2010) found that when unpleasant images were shown to women, their perception of pain was enhanced upon seeing the images. Yet, the research was conducted with healthy women; one can only speculate what the perception of pain is experienced by women who survived wartime experiences, including the direct and indirect effects of war. For example, the South Slavic women's perception of pain might be affected by their mental images and memories of genocide/gynocide, rapes, torture, and violence from the Balkan War (Allen 1996; Baer 2000). How this impacts their oral memory traditions and practices that appears to heal the trauma memories remains to be seen.

War trauma has been found to impact the somatic, physiological, and autonomic nervous systems of individuals and the synchrony of women's cycles (Knight 1987; Mertus 2000; Olujic 1998). The traumatic stress of becoming a refugee or a war crime survivor, and having to navigate uncertain times, can foster feelings of vulnerability (Ogden et al. 2006; Mertus 2000; Totten 2009). These feelings could affect healing properties found in the oral memory process, and being somatically and autonomically intergenerational, may affect future generations since stress is inherited in memory (Campbell 2002; Herman 1992). In all actuality, trauma is a memory disorder.

POST-TRAUMATIC STRESS DISORDER

PTSD has been studied extensively as a result of widespread experiences of the disorder after wartime and other violent events. The Rachel Yehuda (2002) study on the terrorist attacks on the World Trade Center and on the Pentagon reported that up to 35 percent of survivors were likely to develop PTSD, along with various concomitant behaviors, like fear, helplessness, depression, generalized anxiety disorder, and substance abuse.

According to Janina Fisher (2003), autonomic responses, such as increased levels of cortisol and heart rate, become habituated after traumatic events in the following days, months, or years. Memory is impacted along with unfinished neurobiological responses. Mona Lisa Schulz (2005) further explained that traumatic experiences become embedded processes in the brain and body memory circuits, which can then be evoked by a memory that results in physical symptoms of anxiety.

In-depth research on female-specific trauma has not been completed, though historical accounts have alluded to a significant relationship between women's experiences and their biological processes. Searching the archives to 1943, Alfred A. Loeser's (1943) research on menstruation suggests that trauma and PTSD were not distinguished as disorders other than "shock."

In an experiment with four women who were evaluated for possible effects of trauma, Loeser (1943) likened the effects on menstruation to emotional shock as motor and glandular responses, such as emotion to that of sleep.

The four females were subjected to a biopsy, from which specimens showed an endometrium, or lining of the uterus, that had ceased to release hormones due to shock. Thus, these results suggested that shock and trauma do indeed impact menstruation and perhaps other hormonal processes in females. Loeser's (1943) human experiment is one of the earliest known that was in search of trauma variables for females in particular.

Psychological treatment of PTSD has generally not considered the cultural social memories of a victim in the aftermath of violence, though anecdotally, I have found has found that perceiving the past cultural social memories can provide insight and healing for the victim. Likewise, in 1999, Karmin Nader prompted fury in the century's slow and stagnant field of science and memory (noted in Kandel 2006). Karmin suggested that memory is a reconsolidated process that involves, "reactivating a memory, destabilize[ing] it, [and] putting it back into a flexible state" (Kandel 2006). The kolo dance and circles rituals of the South Slavic women may assist in conjuring up these traumatic memories and allowing for them to be defused from the memory system.

We have yet to define a successful methodology for treating PTSD using current approaches. One research study suggests the use of a drug to erase memory in war veterans (a mostly male population). The University of Psychology Professor Jonathan Gewirtz relayed to the press, in defense of his research and the drug, the harsh and difficult memories of PTSD sufferers (Gerwirtz et al. 1997). The erasure of memories as a treatment for PTSD would be culturally devastating to the South Slavic women; those memories characterize the South Slavic-Balkan indigenous way of life. Slavic oral memory traditions do not eradicate survival memory and mechanisms (Anderson 2015a).

Such a gesture would suggest that the oral traditions are shameful, creating a stigma for victims to remember the intergenerational violence, wars, and sexual abuse suffered by their people. Moreover, the body holds memory, according to both South Slavic oral memory traditions and modern neuroscience; simply erasing memories would not reprogram the body from the damage of trauma.

EFFECTS ON MATERNAL PROCESSES

As a hormonal process within the body, female depression has been found to be more acute during menses. Meir Steiner and Teri B. Pearlstein (2000) have hypothesized that there is abnormal signaling to the central nervous system during usual cycles, correlating to findings displaying dysregulation in neurotransmitters, serotonin, and gamma-aminobutyric acid (GABA) (Murray et al. 2008; O'Hara and Swain 1996). According to Anne E. Buist, Kimberly

Yonkers, and Michael Craig (2008) and the World Health Organization (WHO) (2012), mental illness (that is, depression) will be the number one cause of disability by 2020. More importantly, Anne E. Buist, Bryanne E. W. Barnett et al. (2002) underlined that, as the female is the major caregiver for "infants [throughout] infancy, [there is] a potentially highly significant influence both biologically and psychologically on subsequent generations" (101).

In fact, researchers Michael W. O'Hara and Annette M. Swain (1996) posit that there is a genetic contribution for depression perinatally, and premenstrual mood disorders may be channeled through this genetic predisposition toward depression (Borenstein et al. 2003). The latter is in line with the current inquiry about the variables of trauma related to holocaustic genocide/gynocide and the possible impacts to oral memory traditions as shared through future generations.

Thus, for the South Slavic Muslim females who endured war crimes and witnessed war trauma, trauma is likely intergenerational and transgenerational. It has been noted that non-Western traditional cultures, such as in the South Slavic region, tend to have more stable perinatal social support structures, easing the way into motherhood and valuing its role (Murray et al. 2008).

However, with one hundred years of war history, the South Slavic war survivors are vulnerable to not only economic destruction, but also face an internal displacement, which will likely affect the perinatal social support structures available to them, and thus affecting the foundations of their oral memory traditions. Further, the situation may also carry the penalty concerning the gender of infants, displaying an intergenerational trauma transmission (Christie and Pim 2012; Patel et al. 2002).

Stress stemming from maternal-borne fear due to violence and wars etches memory and has been shown to replicate itself in utero (Mertus 2000; Scharf 2000; Schore 2001). "Culturgen" is a term coined by evolutionary biologist Richard Dawkins (1975) as "memes," or the transmission of cultural practices across generations, thus viewing our brain and neurological systems as "cultural consumers" (Campbell 2002, 304). Since culturgens are transmitted through memory and cross-cultural oral traditions, there may be epigenetic transmission of war experiences; there is a relationship between the neurological systems and the physiology of female biology, with stress borne from violence increasing disparities in children's neurological development and increasing the likelihood for mental health challenges later on (J. Fisher 2010; Fosha 2005; Scharf 2000; Schore 2001).

One study found a higher number of preterm births in a group of 5,000 Israeli women who birthed children during the Yom Kippur War (1973), suggesting that there is a correlation between anxiety and the impact of physiological stress responses (McCubbin et al. 1996). Further, a meta-analysis of thirty-seven studies, with some participants matched on menstrual cycle, found variations in maternal care related to cortisol levels, suggesting an epigenetic component to motherhood (Meewisse et al. 2007).

This review of results related to wartime effects on oral memory traditions demonstrates the dire need to further examine how female survivors are affected by war trauma, particularly in terms of biological effects that may impact future generations. A clinical somatic psychological approach to this study provides an ideal framework from which to explore war trauma effects on oral memory traditions.

THE IMPACT OF WAR ON SOUTH SLAVIC ORAL MEMORY TRADITIONS

Within the oral memory traditions, the kolo dance or kolo circle are centered on female biological processes and their daily domestic lives. It is necessary to understand the circumstances under which changes to the oral memory traditions are brought about and the mechanisms involved, such as epigenetics and transgenerational memory practices of those experienced by South Slavic women (Jablonka and Raz 2009). For South Slavic grandmothers in the Ahmica community, the presence of signs and iconic representations serve to help the community to make meaning of trauma; note how the body, the soma, is an integral part of their oral memory applications as a sensorimotor approach (Fisher and Ogden 2009; Ogden et al. 2006).

As a vivid example, an article, headlined with, "After Hague Destroys Srebrenica Evidence, Survivors Feel Pain of Lost Memories," describes the pain mothers felt in not having any evidence or photographs of their missing sons (Deasy and Halimovic 2009). The personal items of eight thousand Bosnian males were destroyed as a part of forensic practice fourteen years after the tragedy (Deasy and Halimovic 2009). One of the Bosnian mothers expressed deep concern about not having a *mezar*, a Muslim grave, nor any of her son's belongings; she reported that it seems as though her son had never existed (Deasy and Halimovic 2009).

The Srebrenica massacre evidence that was destroyed was mandated by the International Criminal Tribunal, causing immense suffering to the many women similar to the Bosnian mother who had no *mezar* for her son. Out of the great incomprehensible loss of the South Slavic women, dignity slowly surfaces through their oral memory traditions (Anderson 2015a; Totten 2009). The Bosnian women survivors of war crimes and war turned to their domestic tasks as a daily art form, a memory-making act to heal. The construction of memory is managed, or at least attempted to be managed, through their oral memory traditions. One must wonder about the impact to the women's South Slavic oral memory traditions.

The cultural practice of South Slavic cup readings is performed in a live contextual archeomythological circle, or kolo, as a part of the reconstruction of social memory (Anderson, 2012a or 2012b; Behnke 1989; K. Wilson 1996). To Bosnian war and war crimes survivors, the cups and the reading of cups in the kolo became the therapeutic framework or space, place, and time to heal trauma in their own communities and families. It stands to reason that the kolo, both the circle and round dance, brings about a sense of space and place for memory. Within the kolo, the domestic arts, and the cup readings, I observed how the past does not constrict the present to hatreds, violence, or intergenerational trauma. For example, gender hatreds, as a preference for sons, are replaced with this somatic psychological reframing and layering of memory.

Oral memory traditions bring forth a voice for the trauma victims whose memories are otherwise silenced and made invisible through blame and shame toward the victims (B. Allen 1996; Herman 1992). Mythic narratives modify old memories and eventually, the pain and the horror are erased by being eased into the South Slavic oral memory traditions (K. Wilson 1996). Those oral memory traditions are solidly based on neurobiological memory processes (Fisher and Ogden 2009; Kandel 2006; Siegel 2008).

CLINICAL SOMATIC PSYCHOLOGY AND FEMALE EMBODIMENT

The intimate relationship between oral memory traditions and traumatic experiences needs to be assessed from the stance of a somatic psychological approach, with attribution to Wilhelm Reich's (1897–1957) early work. Reich revealed the body's ability to remember; thus, experiences, along with structure and class, invoke a collaborative interdisciplinary approach to researching the effect of trauma on our bodies (noted in Hanna 1970; Johnson and Grand 1998).

Understanding the nature of female processes, such as menses, requires a deepened recognition of value in holocaustic trauma research and of women with the prospect of somatic psychological applications as the best fit toward treatment protocols (Caldwell 1997; McCarty 2009; Murray et al. 2008; Schulz 2005). If we review the past thousands of years for the origins of how trauma was healed and how we, as a species, developed evolutionary neurological systems, an integral aspect of somatic psychology, we can better understand how to treat holocaustic trauma cross-culturally and with an engendered perspective (Murray et al. 2008).

Somatic psychological approaches in response to holocaustic trauma are best understood from the perspective of Elsa Gindler (1885–1961), who forged the notion of sensory awareness (Knaster 1996). Gindler suffered from tuberculosis in her young adult years but could not afford to pay for the prescribed treatments. She developed somatic practices based on her readings of breathing techniques, and she employed those practices on a group of Jewish students during World War II, despite the possibility of being discovered and sentenced to a concentration camp. In fact, she continued to develop techniques throughout her life (Knaster 1996).

The application of somatic psychological practices by Gindler identifies the storehouse of treatment resources for catastrophic trauma. But another element is exposed; Gindler's daily life in which culture is manifested. Gindler's situation of treating tuberculosis without funds and her own cultural heritage flowed in a transpersonal model of healing and treatment in which the body/mind was instructional in her traditional setting (Loukes 2006).

Gindler's database of information was borne from her catastrophic illness and the Holocaust in World War II. She did not operate from status quo teaching courses. She focused on aspects of the body, such as breathing and heartbeats, where there had been no previous knowledge or research (Kampe 2010; Knaster 1996).

Gindler went on to work with Heinrich Jacoby (1889–1964), who is known for human learning and creativity in Zurich. Gindler's sensory reeducation, encompassed by her research and body of work, informed somatic psychological practices, especially that of Wilhelm Reich and body psychotherapy—vegetotherapy (Geuter et al. 2010; Knaster 1996).

The same situation exists for this research on trauma and its relation to the oral memory traditions of the South Slavic Muslim female war crimes survivors and war survivors. This study involves the possibility of adding much needed somatic psychological practices for the treatment of trauma, specifically engendered to consider females surviving catastrophic violence (Campbell 2002; Hrdy 1997). Having only begun to explore these field dynamics of female daily life in war and genocide/gynocide requires the inclusion of South Slavic oral memory traditions in this research (Baer 2000; Christie and Pim 2012; de Certeau 1984).

Rebecca Loukes's (2006) accounts of Gindler focused on "daily life" to cultivate breathing, tension, and relaxation practices, and described how Gindler's techniques might be applied to contemporary states of need, such as traumatic events. As such, daily life is the backbone of intangible oral memory practices (living culture) that are especially found in female lives and experiences—basically a collectivizing memory that holds important data informing somatic psychological practices (Van Dyke and Alcock 2003; Baer 2000; de Certeau 1984; Marler 1991).

CLINICAL SOMATIC PSYCHOLOGY AND TRAUMA

Christine Caldwell (1997) termed clinical somatic psychological approaches as the somatic umbrella, making the point of how somatic psychological approaches further develop by "physicalizing them" (17). Caldwell posits that our psychological affective states, our neurological systems, and soma show how embedded our responses are based on what is occurring in our environment. Janina Fisher and Pat Ogden (2009) examined how trauma and psychological effects affect, not just the brain and the mind, but also the body.

Despite decades of research about the relationship between trauma and PTSD and states of hypo- or hyperarousal, attachment disorders, somatoform, and psychoform, Fisher and Ogden suggested that there is an absence of treatment protocols available to directly address post-traumatic psychological effects.

A sensorimotor approach to somatic psychology incorporates somatic interventions that afford regulation of autonomic arousal and promote adaptation and flexibility in response to traumatic experiences (Fisher and Ogden 2009). With the inclusion of the soma and recommendations that sensitivity impacts post-traumatic stress, the authors open the door to research complex PTSD that includes not only associated psychotic disorders, but also female biological processes.

In the book *Trauma and the Body: A Sensorimotor Approach to Psychotherapy* (Ogden et al. 2006), the authors focus on somatic forms as being connected to mental health, a practice and oral memory tradition that spans "thousands of years of practice in the contemplative traditions. . . . [They note that] we have forgotten the hard-earned wisdom of these ancient traditions" (xv). Additionally, Ogden et al. (2006) understand that the interpersonal neuroscience of the brain is wired to connect through a collective lens with other minds and note the importance of mirror neurons to create emotional resonance. In fact, the embedded nature of our neurological system, mind, brain, and soma is an embodied process and webbed relationally.

GENDER-HOLISTIC APPROACHES AND CROSS-CULTURAL STUDIES

According to the International Classification of Impairments, Disabilities, and Handicaps (ICD), it is essential to describe current cross-cultural psychiatry so as to used methods and applications that can be "valid" in each respective local culture (Murray et al. 2008, 423). Much in the same fashion as psychiatric cross-cultural epidemiological research, there is a "surge of interest in culture as an independent variable in design and interpretation of psychiatric research coincides with the spectacular demographic change in the ethnic composition of many developed countries" (Murray et al. 2008, 421). The South Slavic women provide a cultural perspective of trauma and treatment that has not been previously obtained.

Additionally, one of the most compelling aspects of the proposed study is that it is centered on women and does not assume that men's and women's embodied experiences are the same. Current psychological practices do not coincide with women's experiences and may neglect research on the differences between men and women's behavior and somatic movements (Campbell 2002; Mertus 2000). The employment of a gender-holistic approach draws from a data sample that involves the whole of humanity, suggesting that female and males are integrated (Marler1991; 2003; Mertus 2000).

According to scholar Riane Eisler, much of research and history has performed a "massive omission" when not researching females, creating what Eisler termed as "severe inaccuracies" (qtd. in Eddy 2009, 5–27; Marler 1991; 2003). Further, Martha Eddy (2009) stated that, "[the] historical development of the field of somatic education and its relationship to dance points to the omission of dance and somatic education research as a part of marginalization of what I posit as feminine soma and a viable source of data and information" (5). The cross-cultural and gender-inclusive perspective of this research will allow for cultural sensitivity, an approach from which to analyze phenomena so as to identify intracultural elements (Beiser et al. 1994).

KOLO: AN ORAL MEMORY TRADITION

One way in which the South Slavic women have persevered in the face of tragedy is through an intangible heritage tradition in which the interpersonal connection of minds takes place during "kolo," an ancient word for "the wheel" that represents both being in a circle and performing a Mesolithic-aged folk round dance (Christie and Pim 2012, 272–76). The kolo is the circle of information shared with each other, such as skills for healing trauma and sharing life experiences amongst the social collective. The kolo circle format is energy enumerated and organized via somatic movements in their traditional dances and circles from menses and childbirth to harvesting and bees (Christie and Pim 2012; Lockwood 1975; Marler 1991; 2003).

Further, kolo is an oral memory tradition of passing down information and ancestors' knowledge of the body and how to evolve the brain with the layering of new memories through daily life practices. This practice still exists in many modern-day cultures with ancient roots and indigenous people (Van Dyke and Alcock 2003). For instance, the choreographic process of the

Feldenkrais method acknowledges how the dancers are allowed the space and place that facilitate their experiences collaboratively, while transferring cross-disciplinary fields of body practices as embodied knowledge (Ilieva and Shturbanova 1997; Marler 1991; 2003; Kampe 2010).

As a researcher, I experienced the kolo within the collective community of South Slavic women in Bosnia for more than two decades. The South Slavic oral memory traditions, with the inherent foundation of the kolo, are not only an integration of somatic psychological approaches, but also appear to be origins of somatic psychological pedagogical practices (Caruth 1995). With the South Slavic daily life formulating oral memory traditions and organized body movements, there is an ability to extract critical data about holocaustic trauma impacts (Marler, 1991; 2003; Schulz 2005).

The folk circle dances provide female soma information inherent with instructional-educational information, fostering somatic psychological and physical practices (Christie and Pim 2012; Eddy 2009; Geuter et al. 2010; Van Dyke and Alcock 2003). South Slavic oral memory traditions, the body movements of the kolo folk practices created through daily living, are more than adequately qualified as what Dawkins' (1975) termed "culturgen" (Campbell 2002, 304–5).

However, as Judith Lewis Herman (1992) describes in trauma work based on women's liberation movements, culturgen is viewed as the prolonged longevity of PTSD that manifests in transgenerational and intergenerational trauma (118, 120). In other words, trauma memes are passed down through the generation as opposed to cultural practices. Herman (1992) cited a need for a new concept in the treatment of trauma, as "the somatic symptoms of survivors are not the same as ordinary psychosomatic disorders" (118).

Scientists are beginning to provide empirical evidence for information that ancient peoples already suspected to be true. When we are sharing energy and information, there is a two-way experience, the essence of relationships, as in first-person stories, critical data, and survey responses. In the form of the Mesolithic-aged kolo folk dances or its circle, the encompassed energy and information, the basic structure of learning environments, are critical data in research that have unfortunately been marginalized or simply omitted. Herman (1992) acknowledged that complex traumatic disorders have not been fully examined or "outlined systematically," quoting Lawrence Kolb, "post-traumatic stress disorder is to psychiatry as syphilis was to medicine" (Herman 1992, 119). The current study will lessen the gap between understanding PTSD-related effects of trauma and cultural practices.

Given the research, the current study has used the wealth of information embedded in the kolo practices to understand the oral memory traditions shared among the South Slavic women and how trauma has affected their cultural practices and experiences. It is clear that there is a need to further study cultural effects in relation to trauma, particularly given the extant effects on female somatic psychological and psychobiological processes.

References

Ackerman, Courtney E. 2018. "What Is Attachment Theory? Bowlby's 4 Stages Explained." *Positive Psychology.* April 27, 2018. https://positivepsychology.com/attachment-theory/ (accessed March 4, 2023).

Alexander, Jeffrey C. 2012. *Trauma: A Social Theory*. Cambridge: Polity Press.

Alexander, Jeffrey C., Ron Eyerman, Bernard Giesen, Neil J. Smelser, and Piotr Sztompka. 2004. *Cultural Trauma and Collective Identity*. Berkeley: University of California Press.

Allen, Beverly. 1996. *Rape Warfare: The Hidden Genocide in Bosnia-Herzegovina and Croatia.* Minneapolis: University of Minnesota Press.

Allen, Sally G., and Joanna Hubbs. 1980. "Outrunning Atalanta: Feminine Destiny in Alchemical Transmutation." *Signs: Journal of Women in Culture and Society* 6, no. 2: 210–29. https://doi.org/10.1086/493793.

Amoakohene, Margaret Ivy. 2004. "Violence Against Women in Ghana: A Look at Women's Perceptions and Review of Policy and Social Responses." *Social Science & Medicine* 59, no. 11 (December): 2373–85. https://doi.org/10.1016/j.socscimed.2004.04.001.

Anderson, Danica. 2012a. *Blood & Honey Icons: Biosemiotics & Bioculinary: The Pedagogy of South Slavic Women War*. Olympia, WA: Kolo Press.

———. 2012b. "The Transformation from Holocaustic Intergenerational Trauma to Nonkilling Intergenerational Wisdom." In *Nonkilling Psychology*, edited by Daniel J. Christie and Joám Evans Pim, 269–94. Honolulu: Center for Global Nonkilling.

———. 2014a. "Mesolithic Kolo Round Dance, Lagan System and Informed Trauma Practices Tracing the Phenomenology of South Slavic Landscape and Body Movements Inter-Related to Laban Notation System & Informed Trauma Care." *Research Gate* (November): 1–21. https://www.researchgate.net/publication/338298356 (accessed March 3, 2023).

———. 2014b. "The Use of Oral Memory Traditions Embedded in Somatic Psychology Practices by South Slavic Female Survivors of War and War Crimes." PhD diss., Chicago School of Professional Psychology.

———. 2015a. *Blood and Honey: The Secret Herstory of Women, South Slavic Women's Experiences in a World of Modern-Day Territorial Warfare*. Olympia, WA: Kolo Press.

———. 2015b. "The Transformation from Holocaustic Intergenerational Trauma to Nonkilling Intergenerational Wisdom." In *Nonkilling Balkans*, edited by Rifet Bahtijaragic and Joám Evans Pim, 77–104. Honolulu: Center for Global Nonkilling, University of Sarajevo.

———. 2016. "Maternal Fright and South Slavic Oral Memory Traditions: Biosemiotics, Epigenetics, and Somatic Psychobiology Healing Practices." *Journal of Prenatal and Perinatal Psychology and Health*. 30, no. 3 (Spring): 168–91. https://www.researchgate.net/publication/340581143_Anderson_-_Article_MaternalFright2016.

———. 2021. "Spiritual Bonding Impulse Signature." In *She Rises: How Goddess Feminism, Activism, and* Spirituality?, edited by Helen Hye-Sook Hwang, Mary Ann Bevis, and Nicole Shaw, 19. Lytle Creek, CA: MAGO Books.

Anthony, Andrew. 2019. "Interview with Stephen Porges: 'Survivors Are Blamed because They Don't Fight.'" *The Guardian*. June 2, 2019. https://www.theguardian.com/society/2019/jun/02/stephen-porges-interview-survivors-are-blamed-polyvagal-theory-fight-flight-psychiatry-ace (accessed March 6, 2023).

Arango, Diana Jimena, Jocelyn Thalassa Deverall Kelly, Jeni Klugman, and Judith Elena Ortiz. 2021. "Forced Displacement and Violence Against Women: A Policy Brief (English)." December 17, 2021. Washington, DC: World Bank Group. http://documents.worldbank.org/curated/en/593151638940044686/Forced-Displacement-and-Violence-Against-Women-A-Policy-Brief (accessed February 25, 2023).

Asala, Kizzi. 2020. "Lupita Nyong'o's DNA Confirms Humankind Was Born of an African Woman." *African News*. March 12, 2020. https://www.africanews.com/2020/12/01/lupita-nyong-o-s-dna-confirms-humankind-was-born-of-an-african-woman// (accessed March 2, 2023).

Association for Psychological Science. 2018. "How Mother-Child Separation Causes Neurobiological Vulnerability Into Adulthood. June 20, 2018. https://www.psychologicalscience.org/publications/observer/obsonline/how-mother-child-separation-causes-neurobiological-vulnerability-into-adulthood.html (accessed March 4, 2023).

Babenko, Olena, Igor Kovalchuk, and Gerlinde A. S. Metz. 2015. "Stress-Induced Perinatal and Transgenerational Epigenetic Programming of Brawin Development and Mental Health." *Neuroscience and Biobehavioral Reviews* 48 (January): 70–91. https://doi.org/10.1016/j.neubiorev.2014.11.013.

Baer, Ulrich. 2000. "To Give Memory a Place: Holocaust Photography and the Landscape Tradition." *Representations* 69 (Winter): 38–62. https://doi.org/10.2307/2902900.

Bahtijaragic, Rifet, and Joám Evans Pim, eds. 2015. *Nonkilling Balkans* Honolulu: Center for Global Nonkilling, University of Sarajevo.

Baring, Anne, and Jules Cashford. 1991. *The Myth of the Goddess: Evolution of an Image.* London: Viking Arkana.

Barr, Michael D., and Zlatko Skrbis, 2008. *Constructing Singapore: Elitism, Ethnicity and the Nation-Building Project*. Washington, DC: NAIS Press.

Bates, Elizabeth. 2014. *The Emergence of Symbols: Cognition and Communication in Infancy*. New York: Academic Press.

Bateson, Mary Catherine. 2001. *Composing a Life*. New York: Grove Press.

BBC. 2016. "Balkans War: A Brief Guide." March 18, 2016. https://www.bbc.com/news/world-europe-17632399 (accessed March 3, 2023).

Behnke, Elizabeth A. 1989. "Sensory Awareness and Phenomenology: A Convergence of Traditions." *Newsletter of the Study Project in Phenomenology of the Body* 2, no. 1 (Spring): 27–47. https://psycnet.apa.org/record/1995-21416-001.

Beiser, Morton, Margaret Cargo, and M. A. Woodbury. 1994. "A Comparison of Psychiatric Disorder in Different Cultures: Depression Typologies in South-East Asian Refugees and Resident Canadians." *International Journal of Methods in Psychiatric Research* 4, no. 3: 157–72.

Bentz, Dorothee, Tanja Michael, Frank H. Wilhelm, Francina R. Hartmann, Sabrina Kunz, Isabelle R. Rudolf von Rohr, and Dominique J-F de Quervain. 2013. "Influence of Stress on Fear Memory Processes in an Aversive Differential Conditioning Paradigm in Humans." *Psychoneuroendocrinology* 38, no. 7 (July): 1186–97. https://doi.org/10.1016/j.psyneuen.2012.12.01/.

Bibus, Anthony III, and Mary S. Carlsen. 2015. "Ethics and Social Policy." *Global Encyclopedia of Public Administration*. 1–22. https://doi.org/10.1007/978-3-319-31816-5_2402-1.

Blair, Anthony. 2022. "Act of Kindness: Heartbreaking Truth Behind Prams Abandoned at Polish Train Station as Mums Leave Pushchairs for Ukrainian Refugee Kids." *Sun*. March 8, 2022. https://www.thesun.co.uk/news/17879947/prams-left-train-station-poland-ukraine-refugees/ (accessed March 5, 2023).

Bledsoe, Caroline H., with Fatoumatta Banja. 2002. *Contingent Lives: Fertility, Time, and Aging in West Africa*. Chicago: University of Chicago Press.

Borenstein, Jeff E., Bonnie B. Dean, Jean Endicott, John Wong, Candace Brown, Vivian Dickerson, and Kimberly A. Yonkers. 2003. "Health and Economic Impact of the Premenstrual Syndrome." *Journal of Reproductive Health* 48, no. 7 (July): 515–24. https://pubmed.ncbi.nlm.nih.gov/12953326/.

Boxell, Dennis. 2019. "When Serbians Dance." *Folk Dance Federation of California, South*. http://www.socalfolkdance.org/articles/when_serbians_dance_boxell.htm (accessed March 5, 2023).

Briggs, John, and F. David Peat. 1989. *Turbulent Mirror: An Illustrated Guide to Chaos Theory and the Science of Wholeness*. London: Harper & Row.

Brock, Richard. 2017. "The Role of Intuition and Insight in Teaching and Learning Science." In *Tacit Knowledge in Science Education*, edited by Keith S. Tabler and Ben Akpan, 133–42. Rotterdam: Sense Publishers.

Buist, Anne E., Bryanne E. W. Barnett, Jeannette Milgrom, Sherryle Pope, John T. Condon, David A. Ellwood, Phillip M. Boyce, Marie V. Austin, and Barbara A. Hayes. 2002. "To Screen or Not to Screen—That Is the Question in Perinatal Depression." *Medical Journal of Australia* 177, no. S7 (October): 101–5. https://doi.org/10.5694/j.1326-5377.2002.tb04866.x.

Buist, Anne E., Kimberly Yonkers, and Michael Craig. 2008. "Psychiatric Disorders of Menses, Pregnancy, Postpartum, and Menopause." In *Essential Psychiatry*, edited by Robin M. Murray, Kenneth S. Kendler, Peter McGuffin, Simon Wessley, and David J. Castle. 4th ed., 434–50. Cambridge: Cambridge University Press.

Burton, Graham J., David J. P. Barker, Ashley Moffett, and Kent Thornburg, eds. 2010. *The Placenta and Human Developmental Programming*. Cambridge: Cambridge University Press.

Buss, Arnold H., and Robert Plomin. 2014. *Temperament: Early Developing Personality Traits*. London and New York: Psychology Press.

Caldwell, Christine, ed. 1997. *Getting in Touch: The Guide to New Body-Centered Therapies*. Wheaton, IL: Quest Books.

Campbell, Anne. 2002. *A Mind of Her Own: The Evolutionary Psychology of Women.* Oxford: Oxford University Press.

Candau, Joel. 2010. "Shared Memory, Odours and Sociotransmitters or: 'Save the Interaction!'" *Outlines. Critical Practice Studies* 12, no. 2: 29–42. https://doi.org/10.7146/ocps.v12i2.2727.

Carey, Nessa. 2013. *The Epigenetic Revolution: How Modern Biology Is Rewriting Our Understanding of Genetics, Disease, and Inheritance.* New York: Columbia University Press.

Caruth, Cathy, ed. 1995. *Trauma: Explorations in Memory.* Baltimore: John Hopkins University Press.

Cavalli-Sforza, Luigi Luca, and Francesco Cavalli-Sforza. 1993. *The Great Human Diasporas; The History of Diversity and Evolution*. Translated by Sarah Thorne. New York: Perseus Books.

CBS News. 2007. "Bosnian Relatives Shocked by Mall Shooting." February 15, 2007. https://www.cbsnews.com/news/bosnian-relatives-shocked-by-mall-shooting/ (accessed March 6, 2023).

Champagne, Frances A. 2010. "Epigenetic Influence of Social Experiences Across the Lifespan. *Developmental Psychobiology* 52, no. 4 (May): 299–311. https://doi.org/10.1002/dev.20436.

Christie, Daniel J., and Joam Evans Pim, eds. 2012. *Nonkilling Psychology.* Honolulu: HI: Creative Commons.

Clemmons, Jacquelyn. 2020. "Black Families Have Inherited Trauma, but We Can Change That." *Healthline*. August 26, 2020. https://www.healthline.com/health/parenting/epigenetics-and-the-black-experience#A-culture-shaped-by-trauma (accessed March 5, 2023).

Cockburn, Cynthia. 2013. "War and Security, Women and Gender: An Overview of the Issues." *Conflict and Violence* 21, no. 3 (November): 433–52. https://www.jstor.org/stable/24697269.

Collen, Matthew. 2021. "Last Despatches: Why the Balkan Wars Were So Deadly for Journalists." *Balkan Insight.* December 20, 2021. https://balkaninsight.com/2021/12/20/last-despatches-why-the-balkan-wars-were-so-deadly-for-journalists/ (accessed March 4, 2023).

Concept Daily. 2021. "Matriarchy – Concept, History, Examples and What Is Patriarchy." June 11, 2021. https://conceptdaily.com/matriarchy-concept-history-examples-and-what-is-patriarchy/# (accessed March 3, 2023).

Confino, Alon. 1997. "*AHR Forum*: Collective Memory and Cultural History: Problems of Method." *American Historical Review* 102, no. 5 (December): 1386–1403. https://doi.org/10.2307/2171069.

Copelon, Rhonda. 1995. "Women and War Crimes." *St. John's Law Review* 69, nos. 1–2 (Winter–Spring): 61–68. https://www.ojp.gov/ncjrs/virtual-library/abstracts/women-and-war-crimes (accessed March 4, 2023).

Cossu, Caitlyn. 2012. "Yawn and Pass It On." *SiOWfa12: Science in Our World* (blog). September 12, 2012. https://sites.psu.edu/siowfa12/2012/09/12/yawn-and-pass-it-on/ (accessed March 7, 2023).

Cowan, Emily T., Anna C. Schapiro, Joseph E. Dunsmoor, and Vishnu P. Murty. 2021. "Memory Consolidation as an Adaptive Process." *Psychonomic Bulletin & Review* 28 (December): 1796–1810. https://doi.org/10.3758/s13423-021-01978-x.

Cui, Fang, Xiaoxuan Huang, Yiming Jing, Yue-Jia Luo, Jie Liu, and Ruolei Gu. 2022. "How Resource Sharing Resists Scarcity: The Role of Cognitive Empathy and Its Neurobiological Mechanisms." *Cerebral Cortex* 32, no. 23 (November): 5330–42. https://doi.org/10.1093/cercor/bhac017.

Damasio, Antonio. 2010. *Self Comes to Mind: Constructing the Conscious Brain*. New York: Pantheon Books.

———. 2018. *Strange Order of Things: Life, Feeling, and the Making of Cultures*. New York: Pantheon Books.

Dawkins, Richard. 1975. *The Selfish Gene*. Oxford: Oxford University Press.

de Certeau, Michel. 1984. *The Practice of Everyday Life*. Translated by Steven Rendall. Berkeley: University of California Press.

de Mendelssohn, Felix. 2008. "Transgenerational Transmission of Trauma: Guilt, Shame, and the 'Heroic Dilemma.'" *International Journal of Group Psychotherapy* 58, no. 3: 389–401. https://psycnet.apa.org/doi/10.1521/ijgp.2008.58.3.389.

Deasy, Kristin, and Dzenna Halimovic. (2009). "After Hague Destroys Srebrenica Evidence, Survivors Feel Pain of Lost Memories." *Radio Free Europe Radio Liberty*. September 03, 2009. https://www.rferl.org/a/1814205.html (accessed March 6, 2023).

DeGruy, Joy. 2017. *Post Traumatic Slave Syndrome: American's Legacy of Enduring Injury and Healing*. Rev. edition. Portland, OR: Joy DeGruy Publications.

deMause, Lloyd, ed. 2006. *The History of Childhood*. Lanham, MD: Roman and Littlefield.

Doherty, Mary Ellen, and Elizabeth Scannell-Desch. 2012. "Women's Health and Hygiene Experiences During Deployment to the Iraq and Afghanistan Wars, 2003 through 2010. *Journal of Midwifery & Women's Health* 57, no. 2 (March/April): 172–77. https://doi.org/10.1111/j.1542-2011.2011.00115.x.

Eddy, Martha. 2009. "A Brief History of Somatic Practices and Dance: Historical Development of the Field of Somatic Education and Its Relationship to Dance." *Journal of Dance & Somatic Practices* 1, no. 1 (June): 5–27. http://dx.doi.org/10.1386/jdsp.1.1.5_1.

Eichenbaum, Howard, and Norbert J. Fortin. 2009. "The Neurobiology of Memory Based Predictions." *Philosophical Transactions of the Royal Society B: Biological Sciences* 364, no. 1521: 1183–91. https://doi.org/10.1098/rstb.2008.0306.

Eisler, Riane. 1987. *The Chalice and the Blade: Our History, Our Future*. San Francisco: Harper Collins.

———. 1991. "Cultural Evolution: Social Shifts and Phase Changes." In *The New Evolutionary Paradigm*, edited by Ervin Laszlo, 179–200. New York: Gordon & Breach.

Ellison, P. T. 1994. "Advances in Human Reproductive Ecology." *Annual Review of Anthropology* 23: 255–75. https://www.jstor.org/stable/2156014.

Etymology Dictionary. 2023. s.v. "Slavic," January 26, 2023. https://www.etymonline.com/word/Slavic.

Falb, Kathryn L., Claudia Diaz-Olavarrieta, Paola A. Campos, Jimena Valades, Roosebelinda Cardenas, Giselle Carino, and Jhumka Gupta. 2014. "Evaluating a Health Care Provider Delivered Intervention to Reduce Intimate Partner Violence and Mitigate Associated Health Risks: Study Protocol for a Randomized Controlled Trial in Mexico City." *BMC Public Health* 14, no. 1 (July), 772. https://doi.org/10.1186/1471-2458-14-772.

Fehr, Carla. 2011. "Feminist Philosophy of Biology." *Stanford Encyclopedia of Philosophy.* June 22, 2011. https://plato.stanford.edu/entries/feminist-philosophy-biology/ (accessed March 2, 2023).

Fildes, John, Laura Reed, Nancy Jones, Marcel Martin, and John Barrett. 1992. "Trauma: The Leading Cause of Maternal Death." *Journal of Trauma and Acute Care Surgery* 32, no. 5 (May): 643–45. https://pubmed.ncbi.nlm.nih.gov/1588654/#affiliation-1.

Fisher, Janina. 2003. "Working with the Neurobiological Legacy of Early Trauma." Paper presented at the Annual Conference, American Mental Health Counselors. July 2003. https://janinafisher.com/pdfs/neurobiol.pdf (accessed March 7, 2023).

———. 2010. "Brain to Brain: The Therapist as Neurobiological Regulator." *Psychotherapy Networker* 34, no. 1 (January): 1–7. https://janinafisher.com/pdfs/regulator.pdf (accessed March 6, 2023).

Fisher, Janina, and Pat Ogden. 2009. "Sensorimotor Psychotherapy." In *Treating Complex Traumatic Stress Disorders: An Evidence-Based Guide*, edited by Christine A. Courtois and Julian D. Ford, 312–28. New York: Guilford Press.

Fisher, Siobhan K. 1996. "Occupation of the Womb: Forced Impregnation as Genocide." *Duke Law Journal* 46, no. 1 (October): 91–133. https://doi.org/10.2307/1372967.

Fonagy, Peter. 2010. *Attachment Theory and Psychoanalysis*. New York: Other Press.

Fosha, Diana. 2005. *The Transforming Power of Affect: A Model of Accelerated Change.* New York: Perseus Books.

Freudenburg, William R., and Timothy R. Jones. 1991. "Attitudes and Stress in the Presence of Technological Risk." *Social Forces* 69, no. 4 (June): 1143–68. https://doi.org/10.2307/2579306.

Fromm, Erich. 1973. *The Anatomy of Human Destructiveness*. New York: Henry Holt.

García-Muñoz, Teresa, Shoshana Neuman, and Tzahi Neuman. 2014. "Health Risk Factors among the Older European Populations: Personal and Country Effects." *IZA*. October 2014. IZA DP No. 8529. https://docs.iza.org/dp8529.pdf (accessed March 4, 2023).

Gerhardt, Sue. 2006. "Why Love Matters: How Affection Shapes a Baby's Brain." *Infant Observation* 9, no. (December): 305–9. https://doi.org/10.1080/13698030601074476.

Germain, Ellen. 2022. "Why Confronting Holocaust Distortion and Denial Matters." U.S. Department of State. January 31, 2022. https://www.state.gov/why-confronting-holocaust-distortion-and-denial-matters/ (accessed March 6, 2023).

Gerwirtz, Jonathan C, William A. Falls, and Michael Davis. 1997. "Normal Conditions Inhibition and Extinction of Freezing and Fear-Potentiated Startle Following Electrolytic Lesions of Medial Prefrontal Cortex in Rats." *Behavioral Neuroscience* 111, no. 4 (August): 712–26. https://doi.org/10.1037/0735-7044.111.4.712.

Geuter, Ulfried, Michel Heller, and Judith Weaver. 2010. "Elsa Gindler and Her Influence on Wilhelm Reich and Body Psychotherapy." *Body, Movement and Dance in Psychotherapy* 5, no. 1 (April): 59–73. https://doi.org/10.1080/17432971003620113.

Gibbons, Jonathan. 2013. *Global Study on Homicide*. Vienna: United National Office of Drugs and Crimes.

Giesen, Bernhard. 2004. *Triumph and Trauma.* Boulder, CO: Paradigm Press.

Gifford, Terry. 2010. "Biosemiology and Globalism in *The Rapture* by Liz Jensen." *English Studies* 91, no. 8: 713–27. https://doi.org/10.1080/0013838X.2010.518041.

Gimbutas, Marija. 1991. *The Civilization of the Goddess: The World of Old Europe*. Edited by Joan Marler. San Francisco: HarperCollins.

Global Women's Institute. 2017. "Gender-Based Violence Research, Monitoring, and Evaluation with Refugee and Conflict-Affected Populations." U.S. Department of State. September 2017. https://globalwomensinstitute.gwu.edu/sites/g/files/zaxdzs1356/f/downloads/Manual%20and%20Toolkit%20-%20Website.pdf (accessed March 2, 2023).

Goettner-Abendroth, Heide. 2012. *Matriarchal Societies. Studies on Indigenous Cultures Across the Globe*. Translated by Karen Smith. New York: Peter Lang.

Goldberg, Nancy Rule, Jill Mattuck Tarule, Blythe Mcvicker Clinchy, and Mary Field Belenky. 1996. *Knowledge, Difference, and Power: Essays Inspired by Women's Ways of Knowing*. New York: Basic Books.

Goueffic, Louise. 2016. "Patriarchy's Language: Naming Our Species." *PhilArchive*, https://philarchive.org/rec/GOUPLN (accessed February 25, 2022).

Green, Bonnie L., Matthew J. Friedman, Joop T. V. M. de Jong, Susan D. Solomon, Terence M. Keane, John A. Fairbank, Brigid Donelan, and Ellen Frey-Wouters, eds. 2003. *Trauma Interventions in War and Peace: Prevention, Practice, and Policy*. New York: Kluwer Academic/Plenum Publishers.

Greiner, Stephan, Johanna Sobanski, and Ralph Bock. 2015. "Why Are Organelle Genomes Transmitted Maternally?" *BioEssays* 37, no. 1 (January) 80–94. https://doi.org/10.1002/bies.201400110.

Grünberg, Kristi. 2009. "Remembering the Soviet Past in Estonia: The Case of the Nostalgic Comedy 'The light blue wagon.'" *Atslēgvārdi / Keywords* 1: 1–16. http://www.satori.lv/raksts/2560.

Haarmann, Harald. 1997. "Writing in the Ancient Mediterranean: The Old Europe Legacy." In *From the Realm of the Ancestors: An Anthology in Honor of Marija Gimbutas*, edited by Joan Marler, 108–21. Manchester: Knowledge, Ideas & Trends.

Hanna, Judith Lynne. 1987. *To Dance Is Human: A Theory of Nonverbal Communication*. Chicago: University of Chicago Press.

Hanna, Thomas. 1970. *Bodies in Revolt: A Primer in Somatic Thinking*. New York: Holt, Rinehart and Winston.

Hannon, Erin E., and Scott P. Johnson. 2005. "Infants Use Meter to Categorize Rhythms and Melodies: Implications for Musical Structure Learning." *Cognitive Psychology* 50, no. 4 (June): 354–77. https://doi.org/10.1016/j.cogpsych.2004.09.003.

Hanson, Rick, and Richard Mendius. 2009. *Buddha's Brain: The Practical Neuroscience of Happiness, Love & Wisdom.* New Oakland, CA: Harbinger Publications.

Harding, M. Ester. 1997. *Woman's Mysteries: Ancient and Modern.* London: Rider.

Hastie, Carolyn. 2008. "The Spiritual and Emotional Territory of the Unborn and Newborn Baby. In *Birth Territory and Midwifery Guardianship: Theory for Practice, Education and Research*, edited by Kathleen Fahy, Maralyn Foureur, and Carolyn Hastie, 79–94. New York: Elsevier. https://www.researchgate.net/publication/235686259_The_spiritual_and_emotional_territory_of_the_unborn_and_newborn_baby (accessed March 5, 2023).

Herman, Judith Lewis. 1992. *Trauma and Recovery: The Aftermath of Violence—From Domestic Abuse to Political Terror.* New York: Basic Books.

Hershey, Robert, Jennifer McCormack, and Gillian E. Newell. 2014. *Mapping Intergenerational Memories (Part I): Proving the Contemporary Truth of the Indigenous Past. SSRN Electronic Journal* (January): 1–54, ssm.2377486. http://dx.doi.org/10.2139/ssrn.2377486.

Hesse, Erik, and Mary Main. 1999. "Second-Generation Effects of Unresolved Trauma in Nonmaltreating Parents: Dissociated, Frightened, and Threatening Parental Behavior." *Psychoanalytic Inquiry* 19, no. 4: 481–540. https://doi.org/10.1080/07351699909534265.

Hodgson, Geoffrey M. 2004. "Reclaiming Habit for Institutional Economics." *Journal of Economic Psychology* 25, no. 5 (October): 651–60. https://doi.org/10.1016/j.joep.2003.03.001.

Hoffmeyer, Jesper. 1996. *Signs of Meaning.* Bloomington: Indiana University Press

———. 2008. *Biosemiotics: An Examination into the Signs of Life and the Life of Signs*. London: University of Scranton Press.

Homann, Kalila B. 2010. "Embodied Concepts of Neurobiology in Dance/Movement Therapy Practice." *American Journal of Dance Therapy* 32, no. 2 (December): 80–99.

Hopper, Elizabeth. 2019. "What Was the Robbers Cave Experiment in Psychology?" *ThoughtCo*. November 21, 2019. https://www.thoughtco.com/robbers-cave-experiment-4774987 (accessed March 2, 2023).

Horsthuis, Jorie. 2019. "Evidence of Atrocities: Fragments of the Bosnian War." *Politico*. March 20, 2019. https://www.politico.eu/interactive/evidence-of-atrocities-fragments-of-the-bosnian-war/ (accessed March 6, 2023).

Hrdy, Sarah Blaffer. 1997. "Raising Darwin's Consciousness: Female Sexuality and the Prehominid Origins of Patriarchy." *Human Nature* 8 (March): 1–49. https://doi.org/10.1007/s12110-997-1003-9.

Hubbs, Joanna. 1993. *Mother Russia: The Feminine Myth in Russian Culture*. Bloomington: Indiana University Press.

Hubl, Thomas. 2020. *Healing Collective Trauma: A Process for Integrating Our Intergenerational and Cultural Wounds*. Boulder, CO: Sounds True.

Hunt, Lynn, ed. 1989. *The New Cultural History*. Berkeley: University of California Press.

Hurford, James R. 2007. *The Origins of Meaning: Language and the Light of Evolution*. New York: Oxford University Press.

Hurley, Dan. 2013. "Trait vs. Fate." *Discover* 34, no. 4 (May): 48–55. https://docs.google.com/viewer?a=v&pid=sites&srcid=Y2xpbnRvbnZpbGxlLmsxMi53aS51c3xzaG93ZXxneDoxMGVmNWU3YTFkYTk4NGNh (accessed March 5, 2023).

Husslein, Mary Elizabeth. 2013. "The Role of Cognition in Oral & Written Transmission as Demonstrated in Ritual Chant." Master's thesis. Madison, WI: University of Wisconsin-Madison. https://dc.uwm.edu/etd/219.

Iacoboni Marco. 2009. "Imitation, Empathy, and Mirror Neurons." *Annual Review of Psychology* 60 (January): 653–70. https://doi.org/10.1146/annurev.psych.60.110707.163604.

Ilieva, Anna, and Anna Shturbanova. 1997. "Zoomorphic Images in Bulgarian Women's Ritual Dances in the Context of Old European Symbolism." In *From the Realm of the Ancestors: An Anthology in Honor of Marija Gimbutas*, edited by Joan Marler, 309–22. Manchester: Knowledge, Trends & Ideas.

International Criminal Tribunal of the Former Yugoslavia (ICTY). 1995. "Transcript 10 NOV 1995." http://www.icty.org/?cx=006919660147320107200 (accessed March 6, 2023).

Jablonka, Eva, and Marion J. Lamb. 2005. *Evolution in Four Dimensions: Genetic, Epigenetic, Behavioral and Symbolic Variation in the History of Life*. Cambridge, MA: MIT Press.

Jablonka, Eva, and Gal Raz. 2009. "Transgenerational Epigenetic Inheritance: Prevalence Mechanisms, and Implications for the Study of Heredity and Evolution. *Quarterly Review of Biology* 84, no. 2 (June): 131–76. https://doi.org/10.1086/598822.

Jansen, Golie G. 2006. "Gender and War: The Effects of Armed Conflict on Women's Health and Mental Health." *AFFILIA: Journal of Women and Social Work* 21, no. 2: 134–45. https://genderandsecurity.org/projects-resources/research/gender-and-war-effects-armed-conflict-womens-health-and-mental-health (accessed March 6, 2023).

Johnson, Don Hanlon, and Ian J. Grand, eds. 1998. *The Body in Psychotherapy: Inquiries in Somatic Psychology*. Berkeley, CA: North Atlantic Books.

Jones, Brandie. 2021."Childhood Trauma: Signs You're Repressing Traumatic Memories." *Verywell Health*, December 21, 2021. https://www.verywellhealth.com/signs-of-repressed-childhood-trauma-in-adults-5211845 (accessed March 6, 2023).

Jung, Carl G., and M.-L. von Franz, eds. 1968. *Man and His Symbols*. New York: Random House.

Kaitz, Marsha, Mindy Levy, Richard Ebstein, Stephen V. Faraone, and David Mankuta. 2009. "The Intergenerational Effects of Trauma from Terror: A Real Possibility." *Infant Mental Health Journal* 30, no. 2 (March): 158–79. https://doi.org/10.1002/imhj.20209.

Kakissis, Joanna. 2022. "Polish Women Band Together to Give Ukrainian Women Car Rides to Safe Refuge." NPR. April 21, 2022. https://www.npr.org/2022/04/21/1093711322/russia-ukraine-war-refugees-ukrainian-women-poland (accessed March 5, 2023).

Kalof, Linda, series ed. 2012. *A Culture History of Women*. 6 vols. New York: Bloomsbury Academic.

Kampe, Thomas. 2010. "'Weave': The Feldenkrais Method as Choreographic Process." *Perfformio* 1, no. 2 (Spring): 34–52. https://silo.tips/download/weave-the-feldenkrais-method-as-choreographic-process (accessed March 3, 2023).

Kandel, Eric R. 2006/2007. *In Search of Memory: The Emergence of a New Science of Mind*. New York: W. W. Norton.

———. 2023. "Eric Kandel. Eric Kandel Research Interest, Aging, Memory, Neuroscience." Columbia MR Research Center. https://mr.research.columbia.edu/content/eric-kandel (accessed March 3, 2023).

Kashgarian, Asim. 2021. "China Uses Rape and Torture Tactic Against Uighur Detainees, Victims Say." VOA News: South & Central Asia. February 9, 2021. https://www.voanews.com/a/south-central-asia_china-uses-rape-torture-tactic-against-uighur-detainees-victims-say/6201842.html (accessed March 3, 2023).

Katsanis, Sara H. 2023. "Community, Population Health, and Outcomes Genetics and Justice Laboratory." *Stanley Manne Children's Research institute*. https://research.luriechildrens.org/en/community-population-health-and-outcomes/ (accessed March 4, 2023).

Kauffman, Robert B. 2016. "Chapter 2: Psychology of Survival—Who Survives." *Frostburg University*. 1–10. https://www.frostburg.edu/faculty/rkauffman/_files/images_preppers_chapters/Ch02-Psychology_v2.pdf (accessed March 2, 2023).

Kaupen-Haas, Heidrun. 1988. "Experimental Obstetrics and National Socialism: The Conceptual Basis of Reproductive Technology Today." *Reproductive and Genetic Engineering* 1, no. 2: 127–32. https://citeseerx.ist.psu.edu/viewdoc/download?doi=10.1.1.602.3628&rep=rep1&type=pdf.

Kedzia, Alicja, Marek Rybaczuk, and Ryszard Andrzejak. 2002. "Fractal Dimensions of Human Brain Cortex Vessels during the Fetal Period." *Medical Science Monitor* 8, no. 3 (March): MT46–MT51. https://www.researchgate.net/publication/11476257.

Kerewsky-Halpern B. 1985. "Trust, Talk and Touch in Balkan Folk Healing." *Social Science & Medicine* 21, no. 3: 319–25. https://doi.org/10.1016/0277-9536(85)90108-x.

Kida, Satoshi. 2014. "Mechanism for Regulation of Fear Conditioning and Memory." *Nihon shinkei seishin yakurigaku zasshi [Japanese Journal of Psychopharmacology]* 34, nos. 5–6 (November): 117–25. https://pubmed.ncbi.nlm.nih.gov/25536762/ (accessed March 2, 2023).

Kiggins, Sheila. 2021. "Unemployment Substantially Increases Domestic Violence, New Study Finds." PHYS.org. October 5, 2021. https://phys.org/news/2021-10-unemployment-substantially-domestic-violence.html (accessed March 3, 2023).

Knaster, Mirka. 1996. *Discovering the Body's Wisdom.* New York: Bantam Books.

Knight, Chris. 1987. "Menstruation and the Origins of Culture: A Reconsideration of Lévi-Strauss's Work on Symbolism and Myth." Unpublished PhD thesis. London: University of London.

———. 2002. "Language and Revolutionary Consciousness." In *The Transition to Language*, edited by Alison Wray, 138–60. New York: Oxford University Press.

———. 2013. *Blood Relations: Menstruation and the Origins of Culture*. New Haven, CT: Yale University Press.

Knight, Chris, Camilla Power, and Ian Watts. 1995. "The Human Symbolic Revolution: A Darwinian Account. *Cambridge Archaeological Journal* 5, no. 1: 75–114 https://doi.org/10.1017/S0959774300001190.

Kolo Sumejja Women (KSW) War Crimes and War Survivors. Interviews by Danica Anderson, Fear-Transgenerational Trauma. 2000–2022. Last accessed January 14, 2023.

Krug, Etienne G., James A. Mercy, Linda L. Dahlberg, and Anthony B. Zwi. 2002. "The World Report on Violence and Health." *Lancet* 360, no. 9339 (October): 1083–88. https://doi.org/10.1016/s0140-6736(02)11133-0.

Kull, Kalevi, and Ekaterina Velmezova. 2019. "Jesper Hoffmeyer: Biosemiotics Is a Discovery." *Biosemiotics* 12, 373–79. https://doi.org/10.1007/s12304-019-09367-7.

Laber-Warren, Emily. 2015. "Out of Sync: How Modern Lifestyles Scramble the Body's Rhythms." *Scientific American Mind* 26, no. 6 (May–June): 30–39. https://doi.org/10.1038/scientificamericanmind0915-30.

Lafreniere, Julie, Caroline Sweetman, and Theresia Thylin. 2019. "Introduction: Gender, Humanitarian Action and Crisis Response." *Gender & Development* 27, no. 2 (June): 187–201. https://doi.org/10.1080/13552074.2019.1634332.

Lakic, Mladen. 2019. "Wartime Landmines Still Taking Lives in Bosnia." *Balkan Insight*. September 2, 2019. https://balkaninsight.com/2019/09/02/wartime-landmines-still-taking-lives-in-bosnia/ (accessed March 2, 2022).

Laney, Almay, and Allison Bernstein. 2020. "Part 1: What is Transgenerational epigenetic Inheritance?" *Biology Fortified Inc.* (blog). January 13, 2020. https://biofortified.org/2020/01/transgenerational-inheritance/ (accessed March 2, 2023).

Lehrner, Amy, and Rachel Yehuda. 2018. "Trauma Across Generations and Paths to Adaptation and Resilience." *Psychology Trauma* 10, no. 1 (January): 22–29. https://doi.org/10.1037/tra0000302

Levinson, Stephen C. 2006. Introduction: The Evolution of Culture in a Microcosm. In *Evolution and Culture: A Fyssen Foundation Symposium*, edited by Stephen C. Levinson and Pierre Jaisson, 1–41. Cambridge: MIT Press. https://pure.mpg.de/rest/items/item_59302_3/component/file_59303/content (accessed March 4, 2023).

Levy, Daniel, and Natan Sznaider. 2006. *The Holocaust and Memory in the Global Age*. Philadelphia: Temple University Press.

Lienard, Pierre, and Pascal Boyer. 2006. "Whence Collective Rituals? A Cultural Selection Model of Ritualized Behavior." *American Anthropologist* 108, no. 4 (December): 814–27. https://www.jstor.org/stable/4496521.

Lifton, Robert J. 2000. *The Nazi Doctors: Medical Killing and the Psychology of Genocide.* New York: Basic Books; Washington, DC: Library of Congress.

Liu, Yasmine J., Rebecca L. McIntyre, Georges E. Janssens, and Riekelt H. Houtkooper. 2020. "Mitochondrial Fission and Fusion: A Dynamic Role in Aging and Potential Target for Age-Related Disease." *Mechanisms of Ageing and Development* 186 (March): 111212. https://doi.org/10.1016/j.mad.2020.111212.

Lockwood, William G. 1975. *European Moslems: Economy and Ethnicity in Western Bosnia*. New York: Academic Press.

Loeser, Alfred A. 1943. "Effect of Emotional Shock on Hormone Release and Endometrial Development." *Lancet* 241, no. 6243 (April 24): 518–19. https://doi.org/10.1016/S0140-6736(00)43079-5.

Longino, Helen E. 2002. "Subjects, Power, and Knowledge: Description and Prescription in Feminist Philosophies of Science." In *Knowledge and Inquiry: Readings and Epistemology*, edited by K. Brad Wray, 385–404. New York: Broadview Press.

Lotman, Yuri M. 2000. *Universe of the Mind: A Semiotic Theory of Culture*. Translated by Ann Skukman. Bloomington: Indiana University Press.

Loukes, Rebecca. 2006. "'Concentration' and Awareness in Psychophysical Training: The Practice of Elsa Gindler." *New Theatre Quarterly* 22, no. 4 (November): 387–400. https://doi.org/10.1017/S0266464X06000571.

Marler, Joan. 2003. *The Body of Woman as Sacred Metaphor*. Research Gate. https://www.researchgate.net/publication/349993058.

Marler, Joan, ed. 1997. *From the Realm of the Ancestors: An Anthology in Honor of Marija Gimbutas*. Manchester, CT: Knowledge, Ideas & Trends.

Martin, Debra L., and Ryan P. Harrod. 2015. "Bioarchaeological Contributions to the Study of Violence." *American Journal of Physical Anthropology* 156, no. S59: 116–45. https://doi.org/10.1002/ajpa.22662.

McCarthy, Wendy Anne. (2004). *Welcoming Consciousness: Supporting Babies' Wholeness from the Beginning of Life*. Santa Barbara, CA: Wondrous Beginnings of Publishing.

McCubbin, James A., Erma Jean Lawson, Susan M. Cox, Jeffrey J. Sherman, Jane A. Norton, and John A. Read. 1996. "Prenatal Maternal Blood Pressure Response to Stress Predicts Birth Weight and Gestational Age: A preliminary Study." *American Journal of Obstetrics and Gynecology* 175, no. 3 (September): 706–12. https://doi.org/10.1053/ob.1996.v175.a74286.

McGowan, Patrick O., Michael J. Meaney, and Moshe Szyf. 2008. "Diet and the Epigenetic (Re)Programming of Phenotypic Differences in Behavior. *Brain Research* 1237 (October), 12–24. https://doi.org/10.1016/j.brainres.2008.07.074.

McTaggart, Lynne. 2011. *The Bond: Connecting through the Space Between Us*. New York: Free Press.

Meckien, Richard. 2013. "Cultural Memory: The Link Between Past, Present, and Future." Institute of Advanced Studies of the University of San Paulo. June 3, 2013. http://www.iea.usp.br/en/news/cultural-memory-the-link-between-past-present-and-future (accessed March 3, 2023).

Meewisse, Marie-Louise, Johannes B. Reitsma, Giel-Jan de Vries, Berthold P. R. Gersons, and Miranda Olff. 2007. "Cortisol and Post-Traumatic Stress Disorder in Adults: Systematic Review and Meta-Analysis." *British Journal of Psychiatry* 191, no. 5 (November): 387–92. https://doi.org/10.1192/bjp.bp.106.024877.

Meger, Sara. 2011. "Rape in Contemporary Warfare: The Role of Globalization in Wartime Sexual Violence." *African Conflict and Peacebuilding Review* 1, no. 1 (Spring): 100–32. https://www.muse.jhu.edu/article/424034.

Merleau-Ponty, Maurice. 1995/1968. *La Nature: Notes, Cours du College de France*. Paris: Editions due Seuil.

Mertus, Julie A. 2000. *War's Offensive on Women: The Humanitarian Challenge in Bosnia, Kosovo, and Afghanistan*. Bloomfield, CT: Kumarian Press.

Mertus, Julie A., Jasmina Tesanovic, Habiba Metikos, and Rada Boric, eds. 1997. *The Suitcase: Refugee Voices from Bosnia and Croatia*. Berkeley: University of California Press.

Mies, Maria. 1998. *Patriarchy and Accumulation on a World Scale: Women in the International Division of Labour*. New York: Palgrave Macmillan.

Mira, Jose Joaquin, Angel Cobos, Olga Martínez García, María José Bueno Domínguez, María Pilar Astier-Peña, Pastora Pérez, Irene Carrillo, Mercedes Guilabert, Virtudes Perez Jover, Cesar Fernandez, María Asuncion Vicente,. . . . SARS-CoV-2 Second Victims Working Group. 2021. "An Acute Stress Scall for Health Care Professionals Caring for Patients With COVID-19: Validation Study." *JMIR Formative Research* 5, no. 3: e27107. https://doi.org/10.2196/27107/.

Mulder, Eduard J. H., Pascale G. de Medina, Anja C. Huizink, Bea R. H. Van den Bergh, Jan K. Buitelaar, and Gerard H. A. Visser. 2002. "Prenatal Maternal Stress: Effects on Pregnancy and the (Unborn) Child. *Early Human Development* 70, nos. 1–2 (December): 3–14. https://doi.org/10.1016/S0378-3782(02)00075-0.

Murray, Robin M., Kenneth S. Kendler, Peter McGuffin, Simon Wessely, and David J. Castle. (2008). *Essential Psychiatry*. 4th ed. New York: Cambridge University Press.

Murthy, R. Srivivasa, and Rashmi Lakshminarayana. 2006. "Mental Health Consequences of War: A Brief Review of Research Findings." *World Psychiatry* 5, no. 1 (February): PMID16757987. https://www.ncbl.nlm.nih.gov/pmc/articles/PMC1472271/ (accessed March 2, 2023).

National Human Genome Research Institute. 2021 "Epigenetics." https://www.genome.gov/genetics-glossary/Epigenetics.

Nevres, M. Ozgur. 2021. "Perucia, One of the Last Remaining Primeval Forests in Europe." *Our Plant.* November 29, 2021. https://ourplnt.com/perucica-primeval-forest-europe/ (accessed March 2, 2023).

Nickerson, Charlotte. 2022. "Wilhelm Reich." *SimplyPsychology*. March 4, 2022. Last updated February 15, 2023. https://simplypsychology.org/Wilhelm-Reich.html (accessed March 3, 2023).

Niksic, Sabina. 2021. "Survivors of Bosnia Massacre Grapple with Horrors, Deniers." Yahoo News. July 10, 2021. https://news.yahoo.com/survivors-bosnia-massacre-grapple-horrors-061651251.html (accessed March 3, 2023).

Njaka, Ijeoma, and Duncan Peacock. 2021. "Addressing Trauma as a Pathway to Social Change." *Stanford Social Innovation Review*. January 21, 2021. https://doi.org/10.48558/PAH0-0871. https://ssir.org/articles/entry/addressing_trauma_as_a_pathway_to_social_change (accessed March 4, 2023).

Ogden, Pat, and Kekuni Minton. 2000. "Sensorimotor Psychotherapy: One Method for Processing Traumatic Memory." *Traumatology* 6, no. 3 (September): 149–73. https://doi.org/10.1177/153476560000600302.

Ogden, Pat, Kekuni Minton, and Clare Pain. 2006. *Trauma and the Body: A Sensorimotor Approach to Psychotherapy*. New York: W. W. Norton.

O'Hara, Michael W., and Annette M. Swain. 1996. "Rates and Risk of Post-Partum Depression—A Meta-Analysis." *International Review of Psychiatry* 8, no. 1: 37–54. https://doi.org/10.3109/09540269609037816.

Ollikainen, Miina, Katherine R. Smith, Eric Ji-Hoon Joo, Hong Kiat Ng, Roberta Andronikos. Boris Novakovic, Nur Khairunnisa Abdul Aziz, John B. Carlin, Ruth Morley, Richard Saffery, and Jeff M. Craig. 2010. "DNA Methylation Analysis of Multiple Issues from Newborn Twins Reveals Both Genetic and Intrauterine Components to Variation in the Human Neonatal Epigenome." *Human Molecular Genetics* 19, no. 21 (November): 4176–88. https://doi.org/10.1093/hmg/ddq336.

Olujic, Maria B. 1998. "Embodiment of Terror: Gendered Violence in Peacetime and Wartime in Croatia and Bosnia-Herzegovina." *Medical Anthropology Quarterly* 12, no. 1 (March): 31–50. https://doi.org/10.1525/maq.1998.12.1.31.

Omerovic, Azra Husaric. 2021. "Bosnian War Rape Survivors 'Still Afraid to Speak Out.'" *Balkan Insight*. March 3, 2021. https://balkaninsight.com/2021/03/03/bosnian-war-rape-survivors-still-afraid-to-speak-out/ (accessed March 3, 2023).

Ormhaug, Christin Marsh; Patrick Meier, and Helga Hernes. 2009. "Armed Conflict Deaths Disaggregated by Gender." PRIO Paper. October 2009. Oslo: PRIO. https://www.prio.org/publications/7207 (accessed March 6, 2023)

Osborn, Andrew. 2001. "Mass Rape Ruled a War Crime." *The Guardian*. February 22, 2001. https://www.theguardian.com/world/2001/feb/23/warcrimes (accessed March 3, 2023).

Otgaar, Henry, Mark L. Howe, Olivier Dodier, Scott O. Lilienfeld, Elizabeth F. Loftus, Steven Jay Lynn, Harald Merckelbach, and Lawrence Patihis. 2021. "Belief in Unconscious Repressed Memory Persists." *Perspectives on Psychological Science* 16, no. 2 (March): 454–60. https://doi.org/10.1177/1745691621990628.

Oxfam International. 2023. "At Europe's Borders, Migrants and Refugees Are Denied Their Basic Human Rights." https://www.oxfam.org/en/europes-borders-migrants-and-refugees-are-denied-their-basic-human-rights (accessed March 6, 2023).

Parncutt, Richard. 2009. "Prenatal and Infant Conditioning, the Mother Schema, and the Origins of Music and Religion." *Musicae Scientiae* 13, Special Issue 2: 119–50. https://psycnet.apa.org/doi/10.1177/1029864909013002071.

Patel, Priti, Rebecca Wheatcroft, Rebecca Jane Park, and Alan Stein. 2002. "The Children of Mothers with Eating Disorders." *Clinical Child and Family Psychology Review* 5, no. 1 (April): 1–19. http://dx.doi.org/10.1023/A:1014524207660.

Perez, Caroline Criado. 2019/2021. *Invisible Women: Data Bias in a World Designed for Men*. New York: Abrams Press.

Perez, Marcos Francisco, and Ben Lehner. 2019. "Intergenerational and Transgenerational Epigenetic Inheritance in Animals." *Nature Cell Biology* 21 (January): 143–51. https://doi.org/10.1038/s41556-018-0242-9.

Pert, Candace B. 1999. *Molecules of Emotion: The Science behind Mind-Body Medicine*. London: Pocket Books.

Polanyi, Michael. 1948/1966. *The Tacit Dimension.* London: Routledge & Kegan Paul; Chicago: University of Chicago Press.

———. 1962. *Personal Knowledge: Towards a Post-Critical Philosophy.* London: Routledge.

Pollack, Sorcha. 2013. "One Billion Rising: An End to Violence Against Women." *Time*. February 14, 2013. https://newsfeed.time.com/2013/02/14/one-billion-rising-an-end-to-violence-against-women/ (accessed March 2, 2023).

Porges, Stephen W. 2011. *The Polyvagal Theory: Neurophysiological Foundations of Emotions, Attachment, Communication, and Self-regulation (Norton Series on Interpersonal Neurobiology)*. New York: W. W. Norton.

———. 2001. "The Polyvagal Theory: Phylogenetic Substrates of a Social Nervous System." *International Journal of Psychophysiology* 42, no. 2 (October): 123–46. https://doi.org/10.1016/s0167-8760(01)00162-3.

———. 2007. *The Pocket Guide to Polyvagal Theory: The Transformative Power of Feeling Safe.* New York: W. W. Norton.

Ravitz, Jessica. 2011. "Silence Lifted: The Untold Stories of Rape During the Holocaust." CNN, June 24, 2011. http://edition.cnn.com/2011/WORLD/europe/06/24/holocaust.rape/index.html (accessed March 3, 2023).

Religion of Peace. 2023. "What does Islam Teach About . . . Divorce." N.d. https://www.thereligionofpeace.com/pages/quran/triple-talaq.aspx (accessed March 4, 2023).

Remember.org, ed. 2021/2022. "Jasenovac Concentration Camp." Last updated May 4, 2022. https://remember.org/jasenovac-concentration-camp.html.

Reppert, Steven M., and William J. Schwartz. 1984. "The Suprachiasmatic Nuclei of the Fetal Rat: Characterization of a Functional Circadian Clock Using 14C-Labeled Deoxyglucose." *Journal of Neuroscience* 4, no. (July): 1677–82. https://www.jneurosci.org/content/jneuro/4/7/1677.full.pdf (accessed March 5, 2023).

Rhudy, Jamie L., and Emily J. Bartley. 2010. “The Effect of the Menstrual Cycle on Affective Modulation of Pain and Nociception in Healthy Women. *Pain* 149, no. 2 (May): 365–72. https://doi.org/10.1016/j.pain.2010.02.041.

Roberts, Adam. 1999. “NATO’s ‘Humanitarian War’ Over Kosovo.” *Survival* 41, no. 3: 102–23. https://doi.org/10.1080/00396339912331342943.

Roesler, Christian. 2012. “Are Archetypes Transmitted More by Culture Than Biology? Questions Arising from Conceptualizations of the Archetype.” *Journal of Analytical Psychology* 57, no. 2 (April): 223–46. https://doi.org/10.1111/j.1468-5922.2011.01963.x.

Ronström, Owe. 1991. “Folklore: Staged Folk Music and Folk Dance Performances of Yugoslavs in Stockholm.” *Yearbook for Traditional Music* 23: 69–77. https://doi.org/10.2307/768397.

Rosaldo, Michelle Zimbalist, and Louise Lamphere, eds. 1974. *Woman, Culture, and Society*. Stanford, CA: Stanford University Press.

Rose, Steven. 2006. “Eric Kandel: Making Memories.” *Lancet* 367, no. 9524 (May 27): 1721–22. https://doi.org/10.1016/S0140-6736(06)68753-9.

Rossi, Ernest. 2002. *The Psychobiology of Gene Expression: Neuroscience and Neurogenesis in Hypnosis and the Healing Arts.* London: W.W. Norton.

Rotramel, Ariella. 2019. *Engaging Women’s History through Collaborative archival Wikipedia Projects. Journal of Interactive Technology and Pedagogy,* 14, https://jitp.commons.gc.cuny.edu/engaging-womens-history-through-collaborative-archival-wikipedia-projects/.

Rubin, David C. 1995. *Memory in Oral Traditions: The Cognitive Psychology of Epic, Ballads, and Counting-Out Rhymes*. New York: Oxford University Press.

Sarkissian, Alissa Der, and Jill D Sharkey. 2021. “Transgenerational Trauma and Mental Health Needs among Armenian Genocide Descendants.” *International Journal Environment Res Public Health* 18, no. (19): 10554. https://doi.org/10.3390/ijerph181910554.

Schacter, Daniel L. 1997. “False Recognition and the Brain.” *Current Directions in Psychological Science* 6, no. 3 (June): 65–70. https://doi.org/10.1111/1467-8721.ep11512655.

Scharf, Robert A. 2000. “Why War? And Other Burning Questions: An Invitation to Psychohistory.” *Qualitative Social Research* 1, no. 1. https://doi.org/10.17169/fqs-1.1.1121.

Schore, Allan N. 2001. “The Effects of a Secure Attachment Relationship on Right Brain Development, Affect Regulation, and Infant Mental Health.” *Infant Mental Health Journal* 22, nos. 1–2 (January/April): 7–66. https://doi.org/10.1002/1097-0355(200101/04)22:1<7::AID-IMHJ2>3.0.CO;2-N.

Schulz, Mona Lisa. 2005. *The New Feminine Brain: How Women Can Develop Their Inner Strengths, Genius, and Intuition.* New York: Free Press.

Schwartz, Mel. 2018. “Our Quest to Feel Significant.” *Psychology Today* (blog). January 21, 2018. https://www.psychologytoday.com/us/blog/shift-mind/201801/our-quest-feel-significant (accessed March 4, 2023).

Sebeok, Thomas A. (2001). *Signs: An Introduction to Semiotics*. Toronto: University of Toronto Press.

Serón-Ferré, Maria, Natalia Mendez, Lorena Abarzua-Catalan, Nelson Vilches, Francisco J. Valenzuela, Henry E. Reynolds, Anibal J. Llanos, Auristela Rojas, Guillermo J. Valenzuela, and Claudia Torres-Farfan. 2012. "Circadian Rhythms in the Fetus. *Molecular and Cellular Endocrinology* 349, no. 1 (February): 68–75. https://doi.org/10.1016/j.mce.2011.07.039.

Siegel, Daniel J. 2008. *The Neurobiology of "We": How Relationships, the Mind, and the Brain Interact to Shape Who We are.* Amazon Audiobook. http://www.audible.com/pd/ref=sr_1_1?asin=B005OZJFWA&qid=1353880776&sr=1-1 (accessed March 6, 2023).

Silva, Sonia Maria Gomes 2014. "Engaging Touch & Movement in Somatic Experiencing Trauma Resolution Approach." New York: IUGS. https://traumahealing.org/wp-content/uploads/2016/04/engaging-touch-and-movement-in-se-trama-resolution-approach-dissertation-bySoniaGomes-2014.pdf (accessed March 4, 2023).

Simha, Rakesh Krishnan. 2014. "Sanskrit and Russian: Ancient Kinship." *Russia Beyond* (blog). November 3, 2014. https://www.rbth.com/blogs/2014/11/01/sanskrit_and_russian_ancient_kinship 39451.

Simon, Scott. 2022. "Ethnic Tensions Are Mounting in Bosnia-Herzegovina Again." Interview by Frank Langfitt. NPR, January 22, 2022. https://www.npr.org/2022/01/22/1075049588/ethnic-tensions-are-mounting-in-bosnia-herzegovina-again (accessed March 2, 2023).

Singer, Lynn T., Sarah Fulton, Marilyn Davillier, Danielle Koshy, Ann Salvator, and Jill E. Baley, 2003. "Effects of Infant Risk Status and Maternal Psychological Distress on Maternal-Infant Interactions during the First Year of Life." *Journal of Developmental & Behavioral Pediatrics* 24, no. 4 (August), 233–41. https://doi.org/10.1097/00004703-200308000-00003.

Skjelsbæk, Inger. 2016. "Victim and Survivor: Narrated Social Identities of Women Who Experienced Rape During the War in Bosnia-Herzegovina." *Feminism & Psychology* 16, no. 4 (July): 373–403. https://doi.org/10.1177/0959353506068746.

Slapšak, Svetlana. 2005. "Women's Memory in the Balkans: The Alternative Kosovo Myth." *Anthropological Journal on European Cultures AJEC* no. 14: 95–111. https://www.ceeol.com/search/article-detail?id=49519.

Steinberg, Laurence, Deborah Lowe Vandell, and Marc H. Bornstein. 2010. *Development: Infancy Through Adolescence*. Independence, KY: Cengage Learning.

Steiner, Linda, and Barbie Zelizer. 1995. "Competing Memories: Reading the Past Against the Grain: The Shape of Memory Studies." *Critical Studies in Mass Communication* 12, no. 2: 214–39.

Steiner, Meir, and Teri B. Pearlstein. 2000. "Premenstrual Dysphoria and the Serotonin System: Pathophysiology and Treatment." *Journal of Clinical Psychiatry* 61, no. Suppl. 12 (October): 17–21.

Steinmaurer, Gregor, Amela Tahirovic, and Nikola Jurisic. 2021. *Collective & Transgenerational Trauma in the Balkans*. Copenhagen: Pocket Project. https://pocketproject.org/current-projects/international-labs/collective-transgenerational-trauma-in-the-balkans/ (accessed March 4, 2023).

Stiglmayer, Alexandra. 1993. *Mass Rape: The War Against Women in Bosnia-Herzegovina.* Translated by Marion J. Faber. Lincoln: University of Nebraska.

Svoboda, Robert E. 1986. *Aghora: At the Left Hand of God.* Book 1 of 3. New Delhi: Rupa Publication India Pvt.

Tannen, Ricki Stefanie. 2014. *The Female Trickster: The Mask That Reveals, Post-Jungian and Postmodern Psychological Perspectives on Women in Contemporary Culture*. London: Routledge.

Taub, Amanda. 2022. "The Ukrainian Refugee Crisis Is a Women's Crisis." *New York Times*, April 13, 2022. https://www.nytimes.com/2022/04/13/world/europe/ukraine-refugees-women.html (accessed March 2, 2023).

Thanikodi, A., and M. Sugirtha. 2007. "Status of Women in Politics." *Indian Journal of Political Science* 68, no. 3 (July–September): 589–606. http://www.jstor.org/stable/41856357.

Thomas, Nicholas. 2019. "What Are Museums Really For?" *Apollo*. September 23, 2019. https://www.apollo-magazine.com/defining-museums-in-the-21st-century/ (accessed March 6, 2023).

Totten, Samuel, ed. 2009. *Plight and Fate of Women During and Following Genocide.* New Brunswick, NJ: Transaction Publishers.

UNESCO. 2017. "Kolo, Traditional Folk Dance." https://ich.unesco.org/en/RL/kolo-traditional-folk-dance-01270 (accessed March 5, 2023).

———. 2023. Intangible Cultural Heritage. "Oral Traditions and Expressions including Language as a Vehicle of the Intangible Cultural Heritage." January 29, 2023. https://ich.unesco.org/en/oral-traditions-and-expressions-00053 (accessed March 3, 2023).

UNICEF. 2021. "Child Displacement." *UNICEF Data.* Last Updated June 2022. https://data.unicef.org/topic/child-migration-and-displacement/displacement/ (accessed February 25, 2022).

United Nations. 2001. Prosecutor v. Mario Kordić and Mario Čerkez Judgment. *International Criminal Tribunal for the former Yugoslavia*. February 26, 2021. Case Number IT-95-14/2-T. http://www.icty.org/x/cases/kordic_cerkez/tjug/en/kor-tj010226e.pdf (accessed March 2, 2023).

United States Holocaust Memorial Museum. 2011. "The Holocaust." *Holocaust Encyclopedia.* http://www.ushmm.org/wlc/en/?ModuleId=10005143 (accessed March 6, 2023).

———. 2013. "Bosnia and Herzegovina, 1992–1995." Last updated July 2013. https://www.ushmm.org/genocide-prevention/countries/bosnia-herzegovina/case-study/background/1992-1995 (accessed March 6, 2023).

University of California Santa Cruz. 2022. "New Study Shows Transmission of Epigenetic Memory Across Multiple Generations." *Science Daily*. September 26, 2022. https://www.sciencedaily.com/releases/2022/09/220926200451.htm (accessed March 4, 2023).

van Anders, Sari M. 2014. "Comment: The Social Neuroendocrinology Example: Incorporating Culture Resolves Biobehavioral Evolutionary Paradoxes." *Emotion Review* 6, no. 3 (July): 256–57. https://doi.org/10.1177/1754073914523047.

Van den Bergh, Bea R., Eduard J. H. Mulder, Maarten Mennes, and Vivette Glover. 2005. "Antenatal Maternal Anxiety and Stress and the Neurobehavioral Development of the Fetus and Child: Links and Possible Mechanisms. A Review." *Neuroscience & Biobehavioral Reviews* 29, no. 2 (April): 237–58. https://doi.org/10.1016/j.neubiorev.2004.10.007.

Van Dyke, Ruth M., and Susan E. Alcock, eds. 2003. *Archaeologies of Memory.* Oxford: Blackwell Publishing.

van Wormer, Katherine, and Albert R. Roberts. 2009. *Death by Domestic Violence: Preventing the Murders and Murder-Suicides*. Westport, CT: Praeger.

Verdansky, Vladimir I. 2012. *The Biosphere*. New York: Springer Science & Business Media.

Villena-Mata, Darling G. 2022. *Walking Between Winds: A Passage Through Trauma Into Healing*. N.p.: Villena-Mata.

Vlachovà, Maria, and Lea Biason, eds. 2004. *Women in an Insecure World: Violence Against Women, Facts, Figures and Analysis.* Geneva, Switzerland: Geneva Centre for the Democratic Control of Armed Forces.

Vohra, Anhcal. 2022. "Ukraine Mothers Are the Heart of the War." *Foreign Policy*. March 16, 2022. https://foreignpolicy.com/2022/03/16/ukraines-mothers-are-the-heart-of-the-war/ (accessed July 1, 2023).

Volpe, Allie. 2023. "What Attachment Styles Can—And Can't—Explain." *Vox*. February 12, 2023. https://www.vox.com/even-better/23581174/attachment-styles-explain-anxious-avoidant-secure (accessed March 4, 2023).

von Bertalanffy, Ludwig. 1968. *General System Theory: Foundations, Development, Applications*. New York: Braziller.

Wadhwa, Pathik D. 2005. "Psychoneuroendocrine Processes in Human Pregnancy Influence Fetal Development and Health." *Psychoneuroendocrinology* 30, no. 8 (September), 724–43. https://doi.org/10.1016/j.psyneuen.2005.02.004.

Ward, Lewis H. 2008. "Holocaust Memory in Contemporary Narratives: Towards a Theory of Transgenerational Empathy." PhD diss., Exeter, UK: University of Exeter.

Welldon, Estela V. 1992. *Mother, Madonna, Whore: The Idealization and Denigration of Motherhood*. London: Karnac Books.

Wheeler, Wendy. 2006a. "Figures in a Landscape: Biosemiotics and the Ecological Evolution of Cultural Creativity." *L'Esprit Créateur* 46(2): 100–10.

———. 2006b. *The Whole Creature: Complexity, Biosemiotics and the Evolution of Culture*. London: Lawrence & Wishart.

Wilson, David Sloan. 1994. "Adaptive Genetic Variation and Human Evolutionary Psychology." *Ethology and Sociobiology* 15, no. 4 (July): 219–35.

Wilson, Janet Sullivan, Joe F. West, Jill Theresa Messing, Sheryll Brown, Beverly Patchell, and Jacquelyn C. Campbell. 2011. "Factors Related to Posttraumatic Stress Symptomatology in Women Experiencing Police-Involved Intimate Partner Violence." *ANS: Advances in Nursing Science* 34, no. 3: E14–E28. https://doi.org/10.1097%2FANS.0b013e31822724 1d.

Wilson, Keith, ed. 1996. *Forging the Collective Memory: Government and International Historians through Two World Wars*. New York: Berghahn Books.

Winkler, Theodor H., dir. 2005. *Women in an Insecure World: Violence against Women, Facts, Figures and Analysis.* Edited by Marie Vlachova and Lea Biason. Geneva: Geneva Center for the Democratic Control.

Wood, Elisabeth Jean. 2006. "Variation in Sexual Violence during War." *Politics & Society* 34, no. 3 (September), 307–42. https://doi.org/10.1177/0032329206290426.

World Health Organization (WHO). 2012. "Understanding and Addressing Violence Against Women: Femicide." Prepared by Claudia Garcia-Moreno, Alessandra Guedes, and Wendy Knerr, WHO/RHR/12.38: 1–8. https://apps.who.int/iris/bitstream/handle/10665/77421/WHO_RHR_12.38_eng.pdf;jsessio (accessed March 5, 2023).

Yehuda, Rachel. 2002. "Post-Traumatic Stress Disorder." *New England Journal of Medicine* 346, no. 2 (January 10): 108–14. https://doi.org/10.1056/nejmra012941.

Young, Iris Marion. 1994. "Gender as Seriality: Thinking about Women as a Social Collective." *Signs* 19, no. 3 (Spring): 713–38. https://www.jstor.org/stable/3174775.

Young, James E. 1993. *The Texture of Memory: Holocaust Memorials and Meanings.* New Haven, CT: Yale University Press.

Zajicek, Anna M., and Toni M. Calasanti. 1998. "Patriarchal Struggles and State Practices: A Feminist, Political-Economic View." *Gender and Society* 12, no. 5 (October): 505–27. https://www.jstor.org/stable/190118.

Index

adaptive culture, 40
adaptive epigenctic changes, 30–32
Afghanistan War, 83
Africa, 24, 37
African American women, 59
"After Hague Destroys Srebrenica Evidence, Survivors Feel Pain of Lost Memories" (article), 89
Ahmica-Vitez women war crimes survivors, 9–10, 84–85
Allen, Beverly, 83
artifacts, 75–76
Asia, 37
Assmann, Aleida, 28
Assmann, Jan, 28

Baba Yaga, 52
Babenko, Olena, 53–54
Balkan Route, 24, 39–41, 48–50
Balkan War: in Bosnia, 58; children after, 66–67; culture after, 32–33; ethnic cleansing in, 83; history of, 53, 61–62; kolo in, 65; in media, 51; munitions factories in, 1; rape camps in, 83–85; refugees from, 66, 76; sexual enslavement camps in, 36–37; survivors of, 39; tacit knowledge and, 44; Ukrainian War and, 28–29; violence of, 47; women in, 13–14; World War II and, 2, 8, 19, 22, 24, 36, 63
Barnett, Bryanne E. W., 88
Bartley, Emily J., 85–86
Belgrade Serbia, 72
Biason, Lea, 51
biology: bioarchaeological science, 20, 45; biological mechanisms, 36; biological rhythms, 69–72; culture and, 67, 71; epigenetics and, 67–68; female, 15–16, 19, 41–42, 52–57, 86–88; neurobiology, 56, 68; neuroscience and, 7, 14, 81–82, 85–86; psycho-biological processes, 94; in United States, 60–61
Biosemiotics, 56–57, 69
Black Slavery Post Traumatic Stress Syndrome, 58–59
Blood Relations (Knight), 55–56
The Body of Woman as Sacred Metaphor (Marler), 6–7
bonding, 40–41
Bosnia, 1–2, 34, 48–49, 74, 81
Bosnia-Herzegovina, 8–9, 34–35, 52, 58–60
Bosnian Ministry of Works and Social Affairs, 38
Bosnian War, 31–32, 61, 66–67
Boyer, Pascal, 47–48

Brock, Richard, 29–30
Buist, Anne E., 87–88

Caldwell, Christine, 92
Catholicism, 10, 35
cellular memory, 29
children, 24–25, 41, 52, 62–68
circadian rhythms, 68
Clauberg, Carl, 82
clinical informed trauma, 45
clinical somatic psychology, 90–92
Cockburn, Cynthia, 75
cognitive empathy, 14
collateral damage, 81–82
collective memory, 2–3
community, 25–26
compassion, 46
concentration camps, 16, 21, 30, 53, 73, 78–83
Craig, Michael, 87–88
Croatia, 8–10, 74, 78
cross-cultural studies, 92–93
cultural amnesia, 80–81
cultural minds, 41–42
cultural psychology, 9
cultural sociality, 47
cultural traditions, 81–82
cultural transmission, 44–45
culture: adaptive, 40; after Balkan War, 32–33; biology and, 67, 71; cross-cultural studies, 92–93; female biology and, 19; of female social collective, 70; folk matriarchal, 6–7; homeostatic healing and, 13–14; of matriarchy, 33, 45; matrilineal, 33, 35–39; memes in, 88; of Muslim women, 2; oral memory traditions and, 20–21; origin of, 41; reproduction and, 27; in somatic synchrony, 21–22; South Slavic, 6–7, 16–17, 21; tacit knowledge and, 54–55; transgenerational trauma and, 31, 42; women and, 15–16
culturgen, 94

daily life, 91
Damasio, Antonio, 15–16, 47, 63, 75
data analysis, 11–12
Dawkins, Richard, 88, 94
DeGruy, Joy, 58–59
dehumanization, of women, 12
Democratic Republic of Congo, 83–84
denial, 79–80
depression, 87–88
divorce, 44–45
Doherty, Mary Ellen, 83
dual faith-Russian (*dvoevire*), 6–7

ecosopy, 4
Eddy, Martha, 93
Eisler, Riane, 93
elder women, 73
embodied practices, 21–23
Ensler, Eve, 35
epigenetics: adaptive epigenetic changes, 30–32; biology and, 67–68; cellular memory in, 29; of maternal fright, 60–61; memory science and, 67–68; neurobiology and, 56, 68; refugees and, 40; research on, 4–5; of transgenerational trauma healing, 44–46; of trauma, 59–60; war and, 13–14
ethnic cleansing, 83
Evolution in Four Dimensions (Lamb and Jablonka), 15

families, 59–60, 66–67
fathers, 59–60
Feldenkrais method, 94
female biology, 15–16, 19, 41–42, 52–57, 86–88
female embodiment, 90–91
female social collective, 65–66, 70
female social justice: clinical somatic psychology and, 90–92; cultural traditions and, 81–82; kolo and, 73–81, 93–95; for maternal processes, 87–89; for PTSD, 86–87; war and, 82–85

female tacit knowledge approach, 55, 68, 71
femicide, 59
feminism, 34–35, 83
fetuses, 4, 55, 58, 62, 70–72, 88
Fisher, Janina, 92
flesh (*soma*), 6–7
folk matriarchal culture, 6–7
fright/flight response, 74

garbage pickup, 31–32
gender, 51, 59–60
gender-based violence, 20, 51
gender-holistic approaches, 92–93
genocide, 57–58, 73, 83–85
Gerhardt, Sue, 55
Germany, 66
Gewirtz, Jonathan, 87
Gimbutas, Marija, 58
Gindler, Elsa, 90–91
Goueffic, Louise, 15
grammar, 5
Gregorian chant melodies, 57

Haarmann, Harald, 58
Harding, Ester, 51
Healing Collective Trauma (Hubl, T.), 48
healing practices, 57–60
healthy women, 85–86
Herman, Judith, 94
Hershey, Robert, 23
Herzegovina, 8–9, 34–35, 52, 58–60. *See also* Bosnia
hierarchal-patriarchal life, 79
Hitler, Adolf, 28
Hoffmeyer, Jesper, 57
holocaustic trauma, 3
holocausts, 10, 28, 73, 80, 82, 90–91
homeostasis catalysts, 42–44
homeostatic healing, 13–14
housekeeping, 50–51
Hubl, Joanna, 80
Hubl, Thomas, 48
humanitarian aid, 20, 44, 46, 49–50
Humanitarianism and War Project, 81
Husslein, Mary Elizabeth, 57

Ilieva, Anna, 63
immigration, 76–77
informed trauma, 43
institutionalized violence, 32–35
internally displaced persons, 81
International Classification of Impairments, Disabilities, and Handicaps, 92–93
interviews, 35, 53
Invisible Women (Perez), 19–20, 44
Iraq War, 83
Israel, 88–89

Jablonka, Eva, 15–16
Jewish holocaust, 28, 82, 91
Jung, Carl, 69

Kandel, Eric, 28, 65, 68
Knight, Chris, 55–56
Kobiety za Kolko, 66
Kolb, Lawrence, 94
kolo: in Balkan War, 65; in Belgrade Serbia, 72; community and, 25–26; female social justice and, 73–81, 93–95; healing properties of, 64; history of, 21–23; for intergenerational trauma, 90; Kolo Informed Trauma program, 23–24; Laban-Bartenieff system dance movement and, 63; Mesolithic, 7, 21–22, 51, 63–65, 73–74, 93–94; psychology of, 85; research on, 94–95; social engagement and, 25, 27–28; tradition, 7, 11–12, 87; war and, 89–90
Kolo Sumeja Women, 3–4, 32

Laban Bartenieff system dance movement, 63
Lakic, Mladen, 10
Lamb, Marion J., 15–16
language, 6–7, 15, 39, 56–57, 69

LBGQTIA feminist groups, 34
Lienard, Pierre, 47–48
Loeser, Alfred A., 86–87
Longino, Helen E., 55
long-term memory, 28

manmade trauma, 12
Mapping Intergenerational Memories (Hershey), 23
Marler, Joan, 6–7
maternal fright: children and, 67–68; epigenetics of, 60–61; female biology and, 52–57; healing practices, 57–60; oral memory traditions and, 69–72; research on, 47–51, 62–65; social collective for, 65–67; in violence, 61–62
maternal inheritance, 8–9
maternal processes, 87–89
matriarchy, 22, 33, 38–39, 45, 50–51
matrilineal culture, 33, 35–39
matrilineal inheritance, 28–29
Meaney, Michael, 61
media, 25, 51, 74
Meger, Sara, 83–84
memes, 88
memory science: cellular memory, 29; epigenetics and, 67–68; grammar in, 5; memories, 3–5; in narratives, 2–3; neuroscience and, 43; repression in, 77
menstruation, 86–88
mental illness, 87–88
Mertus, Julie, 66, 81
Mesolithic kolo, 7, 21–22, 51, 63–65, 73–74, 93–94
Mies, Maria, 32
Mihailovic, Draža, 78
military, 9–10, 48–50, 64, 83
Minton, Kekuni, 56
mirror neurons, 21–22
mitochondrial DNA (mtDNA), 15, 33, 41–42
modern war, 61–62
mothers, 59–60, 62–65, 67–68, 70–71
mtDNA. *See* mitochondrial DNA
Muslim women, 1–2, 8–10, 30–31, 34–35, 44–45, 57–58, 81–85
mythic narratives, 90

Nader, Karmin, 87
narratives, 2–5, 90
neuroscience: biology and, 7, 14, 81–82, 85–86; of inheritance, 4–5; of long-term memory, 28; memory science and, 43; mirror neurons, 21–22; neurobiology, 56, 68; polyvagal theory in, 15; psychobiological trauma in, 56
nonprofit organizations, 48–49

Ogden, Pat, 56, 92
O'Hara, Michael W., 88
Old Europe, 25, 58
Olujic, Maria B., 51, 83
One Billion Rising project, 20, 46

patriarchy, 15, 32–33, 39, 44–45, 78–79
Pearlstein, Teri B., 87–88
Perez, Caroline Criado, 19–20, 44
perinatal oral memory practice, 56
Pert, Candace, 44
Peter (king), 78
Poland, 66
polyvagal theory, 15, 17, 53, 63
Porges, Stephen W., 15, 53, 63
Post Traumatic Slave Syndrome (DeGruy), 58–59
post-traumatic stress disorder (PTSD), 86–87, 92, 94
pregnant women, 4, 53, 55, 57–58, 62, 70–72
psychiatric research, 92–93
psychology: clinical somatic, 90–92; compassion, 46; cultural, 9; fright/flight response, 74; of hierarchal-patriarchal life, 79; from Jung, 69; of kolo, 85; of manmade trauma, 12; physical pain and, 7; psycho-biological processes, 94;

psychobiological trauma, 56; psychosocial thriving skills, 40; of refugees, 20; repression, 77; of resilience, 13–14, 31; of social memories, 27–28; somatic, 22–23, 28; somatic neurobiological, 2–3; somatic psychological practices, 10–11; of war, 81–82; of war crimes, 8–9

qualitative research, 23

Radio Free Europe, 76
RAM plan, 83
rape, 3, 35–38, 83–85
Rape Warfare (Allen), 83
refugees, 7, 20, 23–24, 39–40, 48, 66, 76
repression, 77
reproduction, 27
resilience, 13–14, 31, 71–72
Rett Syndrome, 68
Rhudy, Jamie L., 85–86
ritual violence, 20
Roberts, Adam, 81–82
Russia, 47–48, 52

Scannell-Desch, Elizabeth, 83
Schoofs, Mark, 16
Schulz, Mona Lisa, 86
Self Comes to Mind (Damasio), 75
"Sensorimotor Psychotherapy" (Ogden and Minton), 56
Serbia, 34–35, 72, 74, 78, 83
sexual enslavement camps, 36–37
Sherif, Muzafer, 14
Shturbanova, Anna, 63
Slavic Moist Mother Earth, 8–9, 42, 50–51, 62, 78
social cohesion, 35–39
social collective, 65–67, 70
social engagement, 21, 25, 27–28
social memories: artifacts and, 75–76; Balkan Route and, 39–41; homeostasis catalysts and, 42–44; institutionalized violence and, 32–35; legacy of, 30–32; psychology of, 27–28; research on, 41–42; social cohesion and, 35–39; tacit knowledge and, 28–30
soma (flesh), 6–7
somatic informed trauma, 9–12, 90–92
somatic neurobiological psychology, 2–3
somatic psychology, 22–23, 28
somatic synchrony, 21–22
Srebrenica women war crimes survivors, 34, 77, 89
Stabilization Force (SFOR) military, 49–50, 64
Steiner, Meir, 87–88
stimuli, behavior and, 55–56
The Suitcase (Mertus), 66
survivors: Ahmica-Vitez women war crimes, 9–10, 84–85; of Balkan War, 39; of Bosnian War, 31–32, 66–67; female biology and, 54; of rape war trauma, 36–38; Srebrenica women war crimes, 34, 77, 89; survival mechanisms, 31; tacit knowledge of, 36; Vagina Warrior award for, 35; of war, 1–4, 6–9, 13–14, 30, 33–34, 42–43, 48, of war crimes, 4, 11–12, 28, 64
Svoboda, Robert E., 22
Swain, Annette, M., 88
Szyf, Moshe, 61

tacit knowledge: Balkan War and, 44; Biosemiotics of, 69; culture and, 54–55; female tacit knowledge approach, 55, 68, 71; oral memory traditions and, 24; research on, 4–7, 75; social memories and, 28–30; of survivors, 36; World War II and, 38
tailored interventions, 3
Talovic, Redzo, 76–77, 79
Talovic, Sulejman, 76–77, 79
Tan, Yi-Fu, 56
terrorism, 86
Thomas, Nicholas, 80

transgenerational trauma, 5–6, 31, 38–39, 42, 44–46, 56
transgenerational wisdom, 47–48
Trauma and the Body (Ogden), 92
trauma healing. *See specific topics*

Ukraine, 7, 23–24, 47–48, 66
Ukrainian war, 28–29, 44
UNESCO, 23, 30
United Nations, 44, 46, 51
United States, 2, 48–49, 59–61, 76–77, 79
University of California Santa Cruz, 60–61

Vagina Warrior award, 35
violence: in Africa, 24; of Balkan War, 47; in bioarchaeological science, 45; femicide, 59; gender-based, 20, 51; genocide, 57–58, 73, 83–85; institutionalized, 32–35; Jewish holocaust, 28; maternal fright in, 61–62; normalization of, 14; rape, 3, 21, 35–38, 83–85; research on, 19–21, 24–26, 79–80; ritual, 20; sexual enslavement camps, 36–37; in United States, 76–77, 79; of war, 16–17, 40–41
Vlachovà, Maria, 51
vodjas, 65
war crimes: Ahmica-Vitez women war crimes survivors, 9–10, 84–85; to children, 62; genocide and, 73; against Muslim women, 30–31; psychology of, 8–9; Srebrenica women war crimes survivors, 34, 77, 89; survivors of, 4, 11–12, 28, 64; Yugoslav International War Crimes Tribunal, 43, 75, 80, 89
Welldon, Estela V., 63
Wheeler, Wendy, 16–17, 43, 54
The Whole Creature (Wheeler), 16–17, 43
Winkler, Theodore, 25
women: in Afghanistan War, 83; African American, 59; Balkan Route women refugees, 24; in Balkan War, 13–14; as caregivers, 46; children and, 24–25; culture and, 15–16; dehumanization of, 12; in Democratic Republic of Congo, 83–84; in denial, 79–80; elder, 73; female biology, 15–16; healthy, 85–86; with holocaustic trauma, 3; humanitarian aid for, 46, 49–50; in Jewish holocaust, 82; LBGQTIA feminist groups, 34; maternal fright healing practices for, 57–60; maternal inheritance of, 8–9; as mothers, 59–60, 62–65, 67–68, 70–71; Muslim, 1–2, 8–10, 30–31, 34–35, 44–45, 57–58, 81–85; in patriarchy, 32–33; pregnant, 53, 57–58, 70–71; refugees, 39–40; resilience of, 71–72; Srebrenica women war crimes survivors, 34, 77, 89; trauma impact on, 19–26; Vagina Warrior award for, 35; vodjas, 65; during war, 50–51; in Yom Kippur War, 88–89
Women in an Insecure World (Winkler), 25
Women Take the Wheel, 66
World Health Organization, 87–88
World War I, 8, 19, 24, 36, 43–44, 63
World War II: Balkan War and, 2, 8, 19, 22, 24, 36, 63; concentration camps in, 53, 82–83; globalization of, 36–37; Jewish holocaust in, 28, 91; oral memory traditions and, 82–83; tacit knowledge and, 38; Ukrainian War and, 44; Yugoslavia in, 78; Yugoslav World War II Jasenovac concentration camp, 16, 30, 78–79

Yehuda, Rachel, 86
Yom Kippur War, 88–89
Yonkers, Kimberly, 87–88

Yugoslav International War Crimes
Tribunal, 43, 75, 80, 89
Yugoslav World War II Jasenovac
concentration camp, 16, 78–79

About the Author

Danica Anderson, PhD, is a social scientist and holds a doctorate in clinical psychology with a specialization in somatic psychology and polyvagal theory. She continues to do informed trauma field work in places affected by conflict, disaster, and war, with more than two decades with the South Slavic Muslim women survivors of war crimes and war . In 2020, her use of Slavic oral memory traditions, a ritual science for the healing of transgenerational trauma, was recognized, and she was vetted into the UNESCO scientific and education council of dance.

Her knowledge that the South Slavs' relations with "the Moist Mother Earth," encoded yet still in the Slavic DNA, in remnants of cultural practices, and especially, in women's everyday constant sustaining of life, is at the core of the healing process. She has experienced the psychosomatic healing that exudes from the women's kolo rituals, and the oral memory tradition science of ancient round dancing and other practices that is not easily captured by traditional empirical methods. She describes it as the women's evolutionary approaches surmounting what most would say are impassable obstacles and arduous struggles largely ignored by those humanitarian and justice agencies that were there to help. In the beginning of conducting informed trauma treatment with the women war crimes and war survivors, she felt that the traumatic experiences and the aftermath in this specific place may serve as a prototype of the planetary situation unfolding presently on a large scale.

Informed by her experience and work across the globe, Anderson has developed her kolo-informed trauma treatments with South Slavic women survivors of war crimes and war, as well as with women in Afghanistan, Africa, Haiti, India, and Sri Lanka. She realized throughout her career that the interdisciplinary fields of science, cultural psychology, epigenetics, and Slavic Studies are invaluable.

The real beginning of her informed trauma clinical treatments started in her childhood. Her parents were World War II refugees, her mother having survived the former Yugoslav World War II concentration camp Jasenovac.

Both her parents became naturalized US citizens. Anderson has authored numerous books and journal articles. She wrote *Blood and Honey: The Secret Herstory of Women, South Slavic Women's Experiences in a World of Modern-Day Territorial Warfare* (2015) and Blood & Honey Icons: *Biosemiotics & Bioculinary* (2012) reaching Slavic people. She currently works with Ukrainian women refugees.

www.ingramcontent.com/pod-product-compliance
Ingram Content Group UK Ltd.
Pitfield, Milton Keynes, MK11 3LW, UK
UKHW041840031026
15587UKWH00002B/906

9 781666 937916